KITCHEN & BATH THEME DESIGN

An Architectural Styling Guide

KITCHEN & BATH THEME DESIGN

An Architectural Styling Guide

by Kathleen Donohue, CKD, CBD

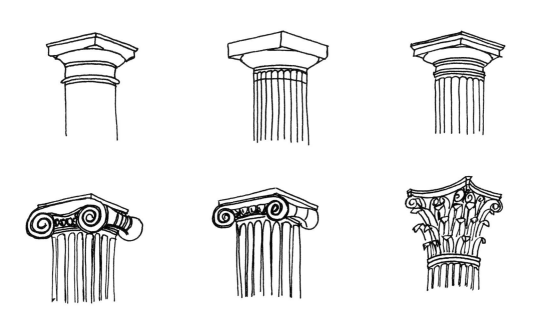

McGraw-Hill

New York   San Francisco   Washington, D.C.   Auckland   Bogotá
Caracas   Lisbon   London   Madrid   Mexico City   Milan
Montreal   New Delhi   San Juan   Singapore
Sydney   Tokyo   Toronto

McGraw-Hill
A Division of The McGraw-Hill Companies

Copyright © 1999 by The National Kitchen & Bath Association. All rights reserved. Printed in the United States of America. Except as permitted under the United States Copyright Act of 1976, no part of this publication may be reproduced or distributed in any form or by any means or stored in a data base or retrieval system, without the prior written permission of the publisher.

1 2 3 4 5 6 7 8 9 0   KGP/KGP   9 0 3 2 1 0 9 8

ISBN 0-07-018134-9

The sponsoring editor for this book was Wendy Lochner and the production supervisor was Pamela A. Pelton.

Printed and bound by Quebecor/Kingsport.

McGraw-Hill books are available at special quantity discounts to use as premiums and sales promotions, or for use in corporate training programs. For more information, please write to the Director of Special Sales, McGraw-Hill, 11 West 19th Street, New York, N.Y. 10011. Or contact your local bookstore.

Other Contributors:

- **Editors:**
  Janice Costa
  Janice Von Brook

- **Home Plans and
  Photography Editor:**
  Annette DePaepe, CKD, CBD, ASID

- **Illustrations:**
  David Bearss, *AIA*
  Kim Leberti

- **House Plan Renderings
  Courtesy of:**
  American Home Styles and Gardening Magazine
  Best-Selling Home Plans
  Donald A. Gardner, Architects, Inc.
  Hachett Filipacchi Magazines, Inc.
  Home Planners, Inc.
  Larry W. Garnett & Associates, Inc.
  The Hearst Corporation

- **Notice:**
  We have made every effort to locate the copyright
  owners of the material used in this book. If an error
  has been made, please let us know and we will make
  any necessary changes in subsequent printings.

- **Cover Credits:**
  Kitchen Designers
    Bernadine Leach and
    Peggy Deras, CKD
  Bathroom Designer
    Thomas Kling, CKD
  Photos by
    Maura McEvoy

PREFACE

Kitchen & Bath Theme Design - An Architectural Styling Guide, presented by the National Kitchen & Bath Association (NKBA®), provides advanced design information for the seasoned kitchen and bathroom professional.

NKBA's intent is to acquaint you with the great potential value that exists in offering specialized design expertise. You will build a strong reputation for yourself and your business as you begin to offer unique theme designs and become involved in the exploration of historic styles in your market.

In the book's first section, Certified Kitchen and Bathroom Designer Kathleen Donohue presents a fascinating progression of American architectural styles in a chronological overview with a detailed discussion of each. It is followed by a discussion of interior styles, and clarifies how to apply specific architectural styles and historic elements in the kitchens and bathrooms that you design by incorporating themes to complement your work.

This book will serve as a tool for inspiration that you can refer to repeatedly as you pursue a more in-depth study of the many aspects of theme design.

> *The philosophy of one century is the common sense of the next.*
> - Fortune cookie proverb

National Kitchen & Bath Association

CONTENTS

PART II

KITCHEN & BATH THEME DESIGN

An Architectural Styling Guide

INTRODUCTION

After mastering the basic skills of kitchen and bathroom design, the next logical step is to develop our individual skills to imprint a personality or character on the rooms we design. We have all studied, in various degrees of intensity, the elements and principles of design, and should have a basic working knowledge of these. However, the ability to create a unique design statement is one that many kitchen and bathroom design professionals believe to be among the most elusive and difficult skills to master.

The prevailing opinion in our society is that creativity and a flair for design are inherited abilities that one either has or does not have. Because creativity is generally regarded as a subjective ability that cannot be measured quantitatively, we tend to be at our least confident when a client asks us about color, fabrics or wall coverings appropriate to the wonderful kitchen or bathroom we have designed for them.

After all, so much depends on personal taste. What if we are merely passing on our preferences and inclinations, with no regard for the clients' unique wants, needs and visions for their homes? Too often, we come across as tentative and insecure when making recommendations about the elements that truly round out and finish our design work.

Although "book knowledge" cannot impart creativity *per se*, it can offer us a wellspring of ideas and mental resources from which to draw on in our search for creative solutions to the design challenges we face daily.

It is in this context that we must view the concept behind the study of theme design, which is to give the designer a solid background in recognizing the elements of various historic design periods that are frequently encountered in residential design work.

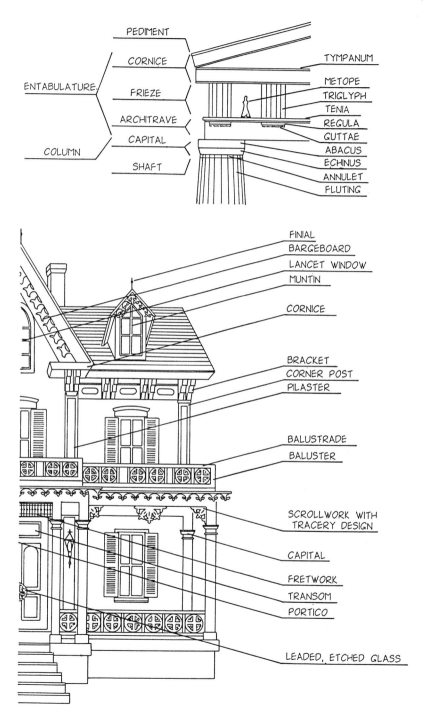

PEDIMENT

CORNICE

TYMPANUM

ENTABLATURE

FRIEZE

METOPE
TRIGLYPH
TENIA

ARCHITRAVE

REGULA
GUTTAE

CAPITAL

ABACUS
ECHINUS
ANNULET
FLUTING

COLUMN

SHAFT

FINIAL
BARGEBOARD
LANCET WINDOW
MUNTIN

CORNICE

BRACKET
CORNER POST
PILASTER

BALUSTRADE
BALUSTER

SCROLLWORK WITH
TRACERY DESIGN

CAPITAL

FRETWORK

TRANSOM

PORTICO

LEADED, ETCHED GLASS

On the following pages, we will attempt to focus on historic periods commonly encountered in American architecture. Obviously, there will be periods that are overlooked. We won't, for example, study Greek and Roman architecture, as we have no common examples of structures dating back to that period, and certainly none that people live in and remodel! However, we will review the classical elements that were borrowed from the temples of Greece and Rome, and incorporated into 19th and 20th century architecture.

By studying housing styles and the historic periods with which they are associated, the professional designer can learn to "read" structures and determine what the overall theme was originally intended to be. Then, by understanding the individual design and material elements that are characteristic to that particular theme, the designer can, with confidence, add new elements that harmonize with and enhance the original design.

A theme, by definition, is the underlying statement that combines separate elements into a unified whole. A theme is a statement, whether whimsical or serious, realistic or steeped in fantasy. What makes a theme design work is the careful balancing of ingredients that enhance or support each other, much like a good recipe blends flavors for taste and character.

Adding an understanding of historic accuracy to your vocabulary will give you the freedom to use familiar and available contemporary materials creatively, with a coherent and thoroughly professional design statement as the end result. Thus, the study of theme design and the understanding of its historic roots can be useful and viable tools for the dynamic designer in today's marketplace.

Over the past 20 years, the kitchen and bathroom business has matured, becoming increasingly sophisticated. Savvy professionals recognize the opportunity for growth and acknowledge the need to keep up with modern interpretations, applications and technologies, lest they find their abilities becoming obsolete.

Studies show that our clients, too, are becoming more educated, sophisticated and demanding with regard to both the quality of our design work and the materials we select to execute those designs. In the past, we could offer one or two cabinet door styles, one hardware selection, a handful of countertop colors and sheet vinyl floor samples, one sink and one faucet, and we were done—regardless of the style of the home for which the kitchen was being designed.

Today, however, those same kitchens and bathrooms present a plethora of opportunities for designers, who are now dealing with kitchens that date all the way back to the time they were remodeled or installed—vintage 1970s!

Today's customers don't want "cookie-cutter" kitchens or bathrooms; they want style. Market studies show that the average consumer is not only more informed, but more confident in making design choices. No longer content to be told what colors and styles are "in" this year, today's consumers choose, more often than not, to surround themselves with colors and styles that make them feel comfortable and happy.

Often, this is reflected in the architectural style of the homes they buy or build. The overwhelming trend in remodeling an older home is to restore the home's original character, and that usually means correcting a previous "remuddling" job, where modernizing and convenient features were added with little or no reference to their immediate surroundings.

The best reason for studying theme design is that it illustrates how to create timeless designs that will age well and blend with their surroundings, giving the impression of always having been there.

The challenge, of course, lies in the designer's ability to incorporate 21st century technology and conveniences into historic period designs so that they work together from both a visual and functional perspective.

Although most consumers appreciate a home's historic or vintage atmosphere, they still expect to benefit from such modern conveniences as a microwave oven, frost-free refrigeration, pilotless ignition for gas ranges, water-saving toilets, steam generators for showers and whirlpools for bathtubs.

Although we may, on rare occasion, encounter a consumer who wants a museum-perfect Victorian home accurately restored down to the last detail, most modern-day families want cable television, computer stations and up-to-the-minute technology in their kitchens and bathrooms.

The bottom line is this: No matter how good the room looks, if it's not convenient and accessible enough to fit the consumer's busy lifestyle, the kitchen or bathroom will not work. The successful and sensitive designer recognizes this, and seeks to strike a balance between form and function to create an environment that is both beautiful and useful.

In his classic book, *A Preservationist's Progress*, author Hugh Howard defines preservation as "the act or process of applying measures to sustain the existing form, integrity and material of a building or structure, and the existing form and vegetative cover of a site. It may include stabilization work, where necessary, as well as ongoing maintenance of the historic building materials."

Few of us will find ourselves involved in true preservation projects, although we may certainly encounter elements of preservation in our work. Mr. Howard goes on to quote the U.S. Department of the Interior in defining restoration as "the act or process of accurately recovering the form and details of a property and its setting as it appeared at a particular period of time by means of the removal of later work or by the replacement of missing earlier work."

Certainly when we encounter "remuddling" on a project, we become restorers when we elect to remove the offending modernizations, such as aluminum sliding windows or an outdated 1960's decor from a stately kitchen.

Finally, rehabilitation is defined by Howard as "the act or process of returning a property to a state of utility through repair or alteration which makes possible an efficient contemporary use, while preserving those portions or features of the property which are significant to its historical, architectural and cultural value."

According to these official definitions, most of the theme design work that we will encounter in our jobs will involve the rehabilitation of older homes and structures, while our work in new construction will be purely thematic.

The essence of good theme design is a strong understanding of the accurate historical elements or language, as well as the philosophy behind it, so that contemporary interpretations can make sense while communicating a coherent theme.

In addition to our examination of historic decorative elements, we will also track basic design principles in kitchens and bathrooms throughout history, and examine how some of our brightest and newest design trends have come full circle. The basics of good design have indeed stood the test of time.

Most important, perhaps, is the recognition that restoration and preservation practices in kitchen and bathroom design make very good business sense. There has been a tremendous growth of interest in designs that are in keeping with the architectural style of a home.

Even in new construction, theme design is growing in popularity, with homeowners using design elements to add character and personality to their homes. The bibliography listed at the end of this book attests to the wealth of material available, and the growing popularity of the concept of theme design. Becoming knowledgeable in the specific roots of your particular regional architectural past is both an interesting and lucrative specialty niche that is well worth exploring.

KITCHENS

Today, it is possible to find examples of kitchens dating back to the 1500s. These medieval relics tend to be in castles, abbeys or similarly official buildings, which may account for the large-scale, multiple-cook structures. The earliest kitchens had to be particularly efficient, since there were no time-saving appliances available to facilitate cooking and cleanup. The use of servants was perhaps the best use of convenience available to most householders in the 20th century.

It was not uncommon to have kitchens divided into distinct work centers, sometimes separated into different rooms. Early colonial kitchens often featured a cook house that was separated from the main residence entirely. In larger, more prosperous homes, safety and problems with sanitation, ventilation, odors and noise usually dictated locating the kitchen in as remote an area as possible.

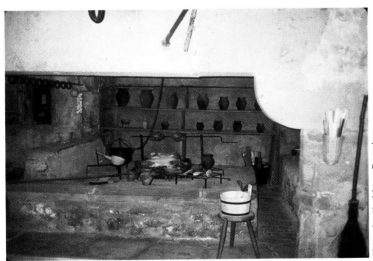

A rare surviving example of a 16th century kitchen located in an abbey/museum in Rothenberg, Germany.

Photo by Kathleen Donohue

Another view of a 16th century kitchen in Rothenberg, Germany.

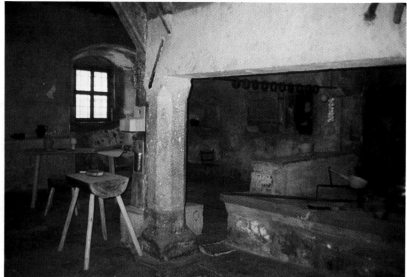

Photo by Kathleen Donohue

Before the existence of electricity, lighting was inadequate at best. Domestic kitchens of pre-colonial times were most often designed around a central work station—usually a large table, with a pantry or larder located off the kitchen. Open shelves, hooks and racks for frequently used items were common.

With the introduction of indoor plumbing, we started to see larders incorporated into better kitchens. The larder, adapted from its British roots, was usually a small room off the kitchen, where water was plumbed into a basin for washing up and gas was piped into a cooker.

Floors and all other surfaces had to be, first and foremost, easily scrubbed. Walls were most commonly whitewashed through Victorian times, after which tiling became a popular option for all surfaces. One of the most significant accomplishments of the Victorians was proving the existence of germs, and the role they play in transmitting disease. This explains the sudden fervor for sanitary surfaces which could be disinfected. Interestingly, this

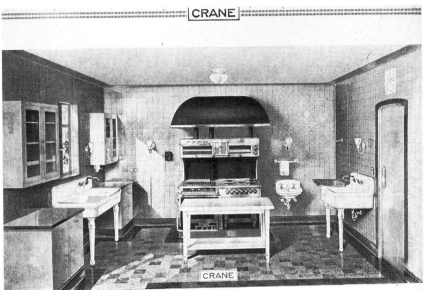

MODEL KITCHEN

Victorian-era middle-class kitchen with butler's pantry (from an early plumbing catalog).

Courtesy of Crane Plumbing Fixtures

preoccupation with germs did a tremendous amount toward promoting regular bathing habits, providing a boost to the use of indoor bathrooms during this time period.

Unlike today, kitchens of the past were not designed for public display. They frequently incorporated a patchwork of different time periods and building styles. However, the kitchens of the past, like the kitchens of the present, were universally accepted as the "heart" of the home. The less pretentious and grand the home, the more people would tend to congregate in the kitchen.

With the turn of the century and the advent of industrialization, we began to see a slight decline in the reliance on servants in the middle-class household. Interestingly, this time period also marked the advent of modern conveniences in kitchens. Fitted cupboards, which allowed for more convenient and accessible storage, began to emerge as an important trend.

The earliest plumbed kitchens usually housed two or three specialized sinks. The open fireplace gave way to the wood-, coal- or oil-fired range, usually a gigantic contraption blackened with oil to prevent rusting. All other surfaces were painted to provide easier maintenance, with ceramic tile being the surface treatment of choice for floors, walls, countertops and sometimes even ceilings.

The predominance of the single-family nucleus became our frame of reference in post-World War II years, and with it came the first university studies that would serve to become the basis for the study of modern kitchen design. Time and motion studies were conducted and scenarios of convenience were concocted to determine more specific information about the average homemaker of the 1940s and 1950s.

Later example showing fitted cabinets and better lighting with linoleum replacing the tile floor.

Courtesy of Crane Plumbing Fixtures

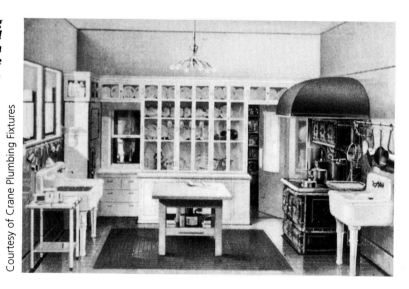

During this time period, the kitchen became an efficient laboratory for the single cook, and the vast parade of time- and energy-saving appliances and gadgets began in earnest. In fact, many of today's kitchen designers were raised in this era, and were schooled in principles of kitchen design dating back to these time and motion studies. Only in recent years has the industry collectively come to the realization that new guidelines for kitchen design were needed to reflect the way we live and work today.

But while much has changed, the kitchen of today is still deeply rooted in the past, having come full circle back to the days when the kitchen hearth was the center of the home: a space used for cooking, eating, companionship and entertaining.

In a tribute to both the past and present, many of today's more modern kitchens incorporate old world charm and features, while concealing modern appliances in period cabinetry.

Today's consumer recognizes that each home has its own style and character, and the kitchen should reflect this. When we skillfully combine vintage furniture elements or period-style casework with modern, efficient appliances, we can create a functional and aesthetically pleasing space that will continue to delight and comfort its users for years to come.

BATHROOMS

Indoor residential bathrooms as we know them today did not even exist until the 1880s. Thus, if the period style you are recreating predates this, you will need to employ artistic license to get an authentic period feel, perhaps incorporating and adapting design elements from that time period that were used in other areas of the home.

Another option is to design the bathroom to reflect a later time period. Does this destroy the sense of authenticity? Not necessarily. In fact, in a true vintage home, the bathroom may reflect a more recent period than the rest of the house, mirroring the time when it was added to the home.

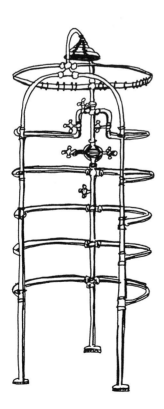

An example of a "needle cage" shower.

The earliest bathrooms belonged to wealthy Victorians, who usually converted a spare bedroom into a commodious bathroom. This practice probably foreshadowed the trend of present-day "empty-nesters" to convert unused bedrooms into fitness and relaxation centers.

By the mid-1850s, finer homes were being built with separate bathrooms designed into them. The fixtures were opulent and numerous. By the turn of the century, a luxury bathroom would be a grand-sized room, outfitted with an enameled tub, shower bath and receptor, sitz bath, foot bath, bidet, pedestal lavatory and siphon-jet water closet. The cost, including all the fittings, trim and traps, could reach in excess of $500. These luxurious rooms would usually be heavily draped and tasseled, and elaborately wallpapered and carpeted.

Interestingly, showers evolved from barracks and gymnasiums, and were most commonly associated with athleticism and men. The shower doused the bather vertically from overhead and was generally considered too rigorous for the "gentler sex." Indeed, it was not uncommon to consult with one's physician before undertaking the experience of the shower bath. In fact, the first home showers were not considered instruments of bathing; rather, they were medicinal aids thought to have therapeutic value in stimulating the proper action of the skin.

As mentioned earlier, the germ theory, confirmed in the 1880s, assimilated into general knowledge in the early part of the 20th century, creating a vast preoccupation with everything "sanitary." Regular bathing and the futility of trying to get clean while sitting in water that became increasingly dirty as you bathed became the topic of many articles in magazines and periodicals of the day.

The state-of-the-art shower became the needle cage shower, an array of multi-nozzle power sprays placed strategically around the body to incorporate a liver or kidney spray, a spinal spray, a bidet spray and a shampoo spray, all with separate controls. A crude valve mixed hot and cold water and passed it through a thermometer on the way to the sprays.

A spacious Victorian bathroom, probably converted from a former bedroom.

Courtesy of Crane Plumbing Fixtures

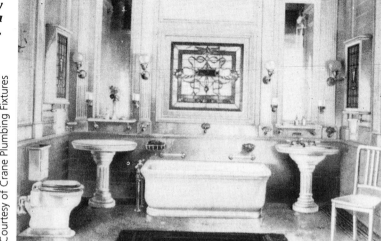

Unfortunately, these valves were not always effective, and the bather ran the risk of being scalded or chilled during the shower. Definitely not for the weak of heart!

The earliest indoor water closets were usually disguised as furniture, much the way their predecessor, the chamber pot, was concealed inside furniture when not in use. Washstands and wash basins were standard features in bedrooms and they translated into plumbed lavatories very similar in form. It is generally accepted that the old habit of using washbasins placed on table tops led to the standardized 31- to 32-inch vanity top height, which we now see giving way to a more ergonomically comfortable height of 34 to 36 inches.

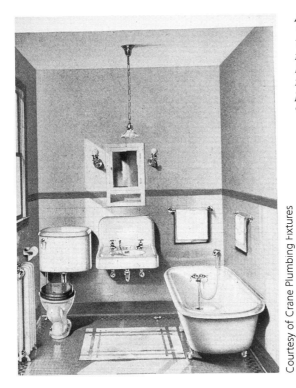

A basic three-piece "bathroom suite." These were the result of the first building codes mandating indoor plumbing in all new construction.

Courtesy of Crane Plumbing Fixtures

A tremendous growth spurt after World War I, which lasted through the 1920s, caused builders to struggle to keep up with the demand for housing. Standardized building codes were adopted and, for the first time, the adoption of indoor bathrooms was required by law in all new dwellings.

No longer an amenity reserved only for the privileged few, the standard three-piece "bathroom suite" became a fixture in new homes across America. These bathrooms were usually minimal in size, with many builders using pre-code plans and converting a closet or pantry for the now-required bathroom. A land shortage in the throes of urban development helped to fuel the trend toward cubbyhole bathrooms, as people traded a spacious bathroom for increased living space. Pedestal lavs disappeared as vanities with built-in storage cabinets became the trend.

According to *Plumbing and Mechanical* magazine, a professional trade publication, "The growth of plumbing in America was phenomenal. In one 25-year period, from 1929 to 1954, sales by distributors of plumbing products and heating equipment rose from $498 million to $2.33 billion, a 367% increase!"

PART I

HISTORICAL SURVEY OF NORTH AMERICAN ARCHITECTURAL STYLES

We see America as an architectural entity when we study all the various styles of homes common to different geographic regions. To help you better understand the origin and thinking of the style periods of the time, the next few pages will explore early homes and furnishings in America, collectively by region.

The Homes of New England

Most early New England settlers lived in dugout cellars or hastily constructed, simple one- or two-room shelters. As they became more sophisticated and began building larger and better homes, they were naturally influenced by the ones they had known in England.

The climate dictated certain elements of construction. Steep, sloped roofs were needed to shed snow, while thick walls were important for insulation against the cold. The kitchen, which acted as the center for most household activities, housed a large fireplace for cooking and heating.

In the early 18th century, copying English Georgian architecture became the style. More attention was paid to detail, with decorative paneling, cornices and pediments replacing the starkness of the earlier interiors. The furniture styles of Chippendale, Adams,

Hepplewhite and Sheraton were used. Trim was painted in vibrant colors, and walls were white-washed with a stippled finish to add color, while maximizing available candlelight.

The Homes of Pennsylvania

The romance of the old homes of Pennsylvania began in the 18th century, when settlers from Germany, Switzerland, Scotland, Ireland and England brought their Folk designs to the land of William Penn. Squared logs, native stone and brick were all used, although, when we think of a typical Pennsylvania home, the rugged and beautiful stone buildings naturally come to mind.

Modest decoration was the rule, partly because of religious beliefs which held simplicity to be a virtue; however, the love of color showed through in interior decoration.

Colorful Dutch tiles imported from Holland were used on walls as well as around fireplaces and hearths. One house might have tan woodwork, red cupboard interiors and black baseboards; another might sport dark green ceilings edged in mustard yellow woodwork. Paneling and trim were frequently beaded.

The land of Pennsylvania was bountiful in its supply of both building materials and food, and the settlers brought along a wealth of diversity in terms of personal experiences, ethnic backgrounds and beliefs. The diversity of the people was reflected in the many examples of true folk architecture, which remained rich in variety and rugged elegance.

The Homes of the Cities

Housing was desperately needed in the wake of the American Revolution, which left the country devastated. The Federal-style row houses (copied from pattern books drawn by British architects) proliferated throughout the colonies between 1783 and 1825, and proved that, while the revolution had been political, it had never been cultural.

The designs utilized classical forms, with Adams, Hepplewhite, Sheraton, Regency and Directoire furniture becoming popular. Colors progressed along with furniture styles, from pastels during the Adams period to strong, solid colors during the Regency and Directoire periods. A feeling of heaviness and solidity prevailed.

From 1825 on, the history of our nation and the influence of the world upon it can be chronicled by its rapidly changing architecture; almost each successive decade produced a new style. The ensuing architectural medley progressed from stately Greek Revival and Gothic Revival through the nostalgic romanticism of the Picturesque styles at the turn of the century.

The Federal style of architecture featured in row housing became the style of the day, popular with rich and poor alike. Evidence of wealth was all but invisible from the outside, becoming evident only in the homes' interiors.

Since architects were virtually nonexistent, clusters of homes sprang up, built on speculation by builders who copied the style from existing pattern books.

The established dimensions of these early 19th century dwellings were to remain somewhat unchanged until the last quarter of the century. Typically, they were 20 to 25 feet wide and, for the sake of proper ventilation and light, only two rooms deep.

The Homes of the South

While visiting the Southern seaboard, George Washington was quoted as saying, "The land is low and swampy and not well suited for growing food crops. Mosquitoes by the thousands rise from the swamps and marshes."

Ironically, though, the people of the Tidewater region not only lived and prospered there, but ushered in an era of splendor in architecture. This region, which was comprised of the states of Virginia, Maryland, Georgia and the Carolinas, became the habitat of a comparatively wealthy population. Virginia, the richest of the colonies, could afford to put up buildings that were prime examples of the latest taste, and were good examples of the spreading Georgian and Greek Revival styles.

A typical Southern version of the Georgian house is Mount Vernon, with its beautifully proportioned, brick-structured portico and its stately columns.

Inside such a house, gleaming furniture reflected the candlelight from crystal chandeliers. Tapestries, mirrors and paintings glowed on paneled walls. White and pastel colors were commonly used, while the furniture of Queen Anne, Chippendale and Hepplewhite was favored. An interest in the opulence of French design was evident, yet it was subdued by the neo-classical lines of our strong English heritage.

The Homes of the Midwest

The agricultural heartland formed a vital thread in the weaving of a new country. Its settlers were adventurers from the Eastern seaboard or immigrants just off the boats from Europe. They came by flatboat or wagon, carefully moving their few precious possessions while struggling with unfamiliar territory and hardships.

The privations passed quickly and the Midwest was soon a prosperous area. Its vitality was expressed in a variety of architectural styles. Frank Lloyd Wright designed houses which were said to be "the first truly democratic expressions of our democracy."

Tudor houses, built around the turn of the century, were part of the Gothic Revival, which grew up in America in the 19th century. These homes were etched deeply into the souls of the English people, and, consequently, had meaning for their American descendants. American versions were often massive, sprawling structures, clothed in the stylistic skins of their antecedents. Robust timbers decorated their gabled exteriors, creating panels filled in with either plaster or brickwork.

Windows were leaded, and frequently featured small, diamond-shaped panes called "quarries." There was usually a bay window, considered the most striking feature of English residential architecture.

Front doors opened into large, wainscoted hallways with tiled floors. In the living rooms, oak paneling often covered the walls, and decorative plaster ceilings displayed the Tudor Rose.

Where walls joined the ceilings, intricately carved moldings were fixed. The skills of talented craftsmen came to light again through the ornate fireplaces, which often projected outward, forming arched alcoves on either side.

The Homes of the Far West

At the time of our country's birth, the Far West was but a colonial possession of Spain, inhabited largely by Mexican and American natives. Much of the Spanish architecture of the West reflects the influence of the early inhabitants. The Spaniards found the adobe, stone and wood structures of the Mexican natives ideal for the climate, and they adapted these simple designs to their own lifestyles. What emerged is called Mission or Southwest style, characterized by heavy plastered adobe brick walls, ceramic tile, warm earth colors and a predominance of geometric patterns.

The discovery of gold in the 1840s brought in thousands of pioneers, literally overnight, lured by tales of instant wealth. Following these fortune seekers came settlers who possessed fond memories of their former clean-cut, wood-frame New England homes. The Western ranch house blends both styles.

Urban expansion in the late 19th century gave birth to the Western Palace, typified today by the ornate Victorian row houses of San Francisco, with their beautiful bay windows.

The invention of steam-powered woodworking machinery added impetus to the Victorian craze for ornamental detail, and great quantities of moldings, scrolls and other embellishments were mass produced to adorn facades, in what came to be called "carpenter" Gothic.

Comprehending the initial classification of the American house is imperative to understanding not only the tradition of the design, but of the people who inhabited these homes over the centuries. The story of our homes is the story of our nation.

And so we begin to understand what American design tradition is all about.

Architectural Home Styles

What follows is a study of architectural home styles and a description of the typical interiors which could be found within them.

Establishing a theme for the space helps the designer organize the project. Once a definite style is identified, many choices are automatically eliminated; therefore, a more manageable range of choices can be presented to the client.

Kitchen designers often wonder, *How do I know what is appropriate for a specific architectural style?* The question is difficult to answer because there are few guidelines to follow. Many architectural periods have distinctive furniture styles, but they had no kitchens for us to study, therefore, we must adapt furniture to cabinetry. We must also contend with the functional limitations of modern appliances.

To successfully create a room reminiscent of the past, designers should strive to create the feeling of the requested style, rather than an actual reproduction of the craftsmanship of the period.

To accomplish this aspect of theme style design, kitchen designers must first understand architecture; second, be familiar with the furniture, styles and fashions of each era; and third, translate this information into an acceptable modern kitchen with the appropriate period motif. It is a challenge well worth the effort for the true professional in the kitchen and bathroom industry.

This section will attempt to identify original architectural housing styles and then show you an example of a contemporary interpretation from housing being built today.

New home plans are shown here to assist you in understanding how architectural home styles have evolved.

English and Dutch Colonial
1650 - 1750

Among the first homes to be built in the colonies, the English and Dutch Colonials built during this period were modest, low-ceilinged homes with small windows. These structures were simple and medieval-styled, typically taking up a single story, with little or no overhang on the sides.

The flared eaves are typical of the Dutch Colonial style while the straight eaves are English Colonial.

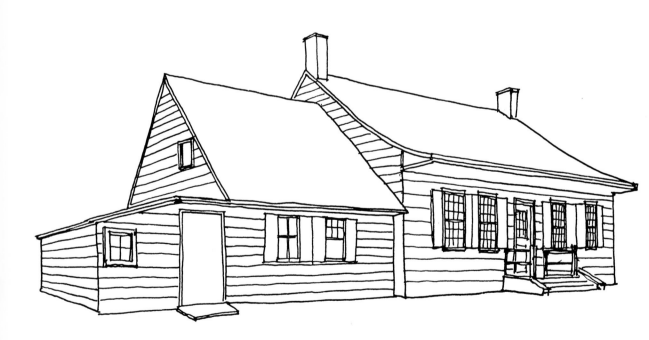

English and Dutch influence was most predominant, with a large, central chimney playing an important role in colder New England climates. English Colonials typically had straight eaves, while Dutch Colonials had eaves that curved out or slightly upward at the cornices. Although influenced by European models dating back to the Middle Ages, with posts and beams and pegged connections, the homes were adapted to suit local conditions, with construction and design being adapted where necessary to make use of the materials at hand.

The typical 17th century colonial house was generally cramped and crowded. It was not uncommon to find extended families of 10 or 12 people living together. The privacy that we take for granted today was virtually unknown during this era.

The Puritans took great pride in their homes, and relished bright colors. Furniture, which included storage chests, trestle tables, gate-leg tables, rush-seated stools and benches, was painted or stenciled. Cabinetry consisted of free-standing cupboards that were rare and elaborate show pieces, designed to house clay pitchers, pots, slipware and wooden plates. Pewter and silver pieces were also displayed.

Fabrics were used primarily as bed hangings, upholstery and wall hangings. They were not used to cover windows, which were usually shuttered. Red, yellow and dark green woolens and linens were popular, but quilted fabrics and lots of homespun materials were also common. Moldings and furniture were painted with milkpaints—raw paint pigment mixed with skimmed milk—instead of oil or water. Pine paneling and wide-plank pine floors were left natural and scrubbed with sand until they were velvety-smooth. Walls that were not paneled were often plastered to ensure smoothness.

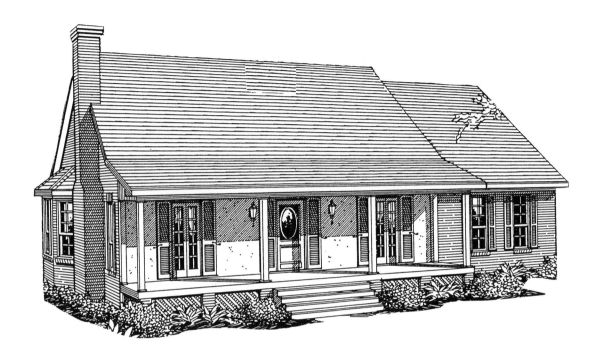

Modern interpretation of an early Dutch Colonial style.
The bay window and full porch are modern additions.

A contemporary example of a rambling Early Colonial style.
True Colonials are much more simple and rustic.

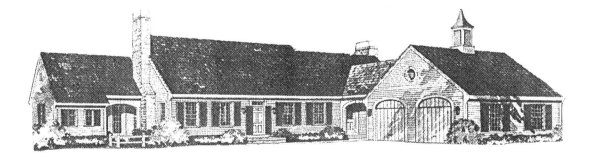

A typical Georgian "salt box" style home with clapboard siding, symmetrical window alignment and heavy ornamentation over doors and windows.

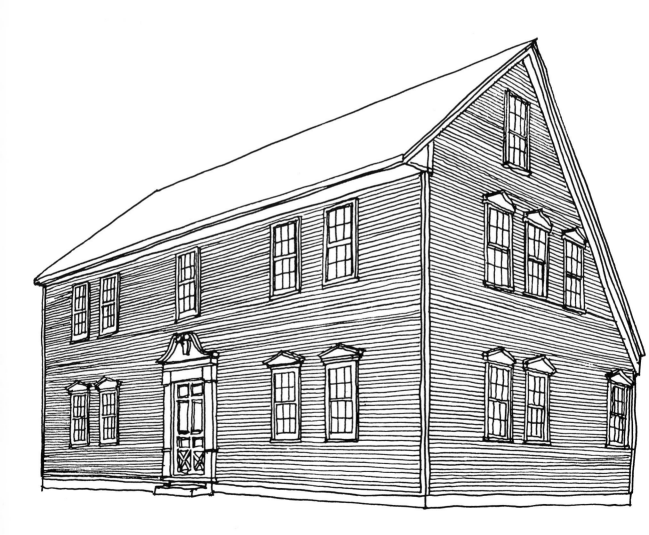

Georgian and Adams
1730 - 1820

Most Georgian homes were at least two stories high, featuring a symmetrical design. The front entrance was typically centered and trimmed with a decorative crown or triangular pediment, and flanked by columns or pilaster supports. Six to 12-pane double-hung windows were aligned vertically and horizontally.

This Georgian-inspired adaptation features a Palladian-style window and an elaborate porch that would be more typical of Greek Revival.

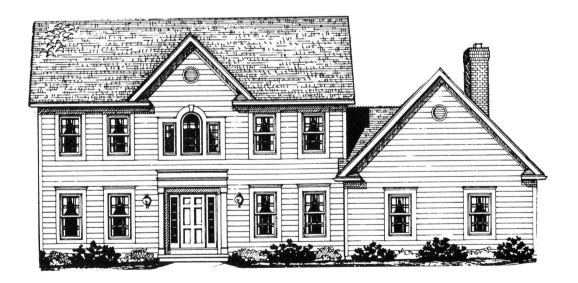

Tooth-like dentil molding often ornamented the cornices. Central chimneys were typical in the Northeast climates, while in the South, they tended to be paired at the ends of the homes. The later Adams style had very similar characteristics to the Georgian, with more refined features and added ornamentation.

A modern interpretation of Georgian with brick exterior, dentil molding and symmetrical alignment of windows. Pilasters adorn entrance and box bay window.

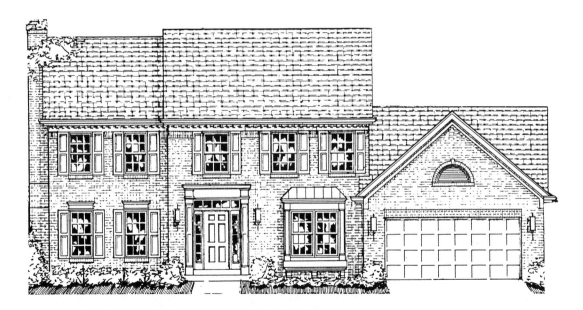

The influence of classical architecture dates back to the work of the 16th century Italian architect Andrea Palladio, who studied the ruins of Roman temples and interpreted them into rules of proportion and scale, combining elements of the sacred with those of the domestic, using a temple facade on villas and palaces. With study and careful

Symmetrical dormers, elaborate door pediment and gable-end chimneys help to define this contemporary interpretation as Georgian and Adams in influence.

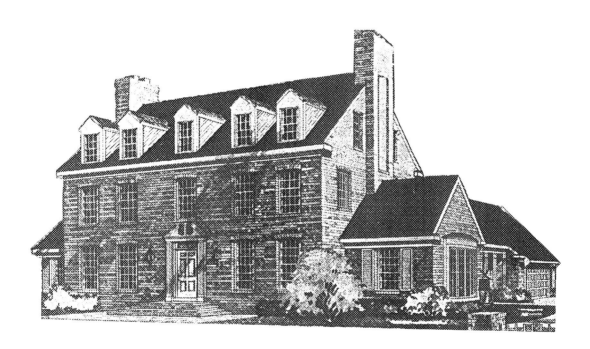

application, Palladio defined the vocabulary of architecture developed in ancient Rome. He believed that by employing that vocabulary properly, one could produce beautiful buildings. Palladio claimed that arithmetical calculations could be used to achieve architectural harmony. His theory, in short, was this: "Reduce it to design."

Inigo Jones, a 17th century English architect, was greatly influenced by Palladio. Jones also traveled to Rome to study classical architectural elements.

Two 18th century architects, Robert and James Adams, were heirs to this tradition. However, the Adams brothers softened some of the more rigid rules, moving toward a freer interpretation of the classical sources. The brothers published a classic book, *Works in Architecture*, which was later sold in smaller and cheaper editions, leading the way to the popular "pattern books" of the times.

The result of all this was a standardized method of balancing the proportional widths and heights of columns and cornices and other shapes in design. In fact, many architectural historians have traced specific architectural elements in existing houses back to the pattern books of the era. For instance, moldings are of great importance in the Georgian house. A classical Palladian wall consists of specific parts that relate back to Roman columns. Topped by a cornice mold at the ceiling, with a secondary band of molding immediately below, called a frieze, the upper half of the wall is called the infill, which could be plastered, paneled or papered.

The wall is divided more or less in half by a molding called a chair rail. The wall section below the chair rail is called the dado, and was most often made from painted paneling. An elaborate base mold would mimic the base of a column. Repeat designs on cornices and friezes would be dentil, egg and dart, Greek key, acanthus leaf, Vitruvian scroll or bay leaf garland patterns.

Rich mahogany, or woods stained to imitate it, would be used as moldings, paneling and flooring. Windows would be festooned and draped with damasks fashioned in vibrant colors.

The 18th century saw a tremendous enthusiasm for everything Chinese, and many English and American furniture makers met this demand by developing a "Chinoiserie" decorative style, with Chippendale being the most recognizable example of this. Willow pattern china, porcelain figurines, delftware, landscape paintings and portraits adorned Georgian rooms. "Queen Anne" tables and chairs were typical, featuring the animal-like "cabriole" French leg or ball-and-claw feet. A well-defined system was practiced where colors were used to contrast with one another, rather than to match. White paint was used to enliven and highlight moldings.

The later Adams style illustrates a reawakening of interest in classical themes, such as Roman, Greek and Etruscan. Colors were softened to pale greens, blues and pinks. Moldings become slightly less massive, their designs more delicate and intricate.

Adams ceilings were ornamented with elaborate plaster decorations in the more important and public rooms. In fact, Hepplewhite, Sheraton and Duncan Phyfe, the American counterparts of these famous English furniture designers, still display classical ornamentation and form, although they are lighter and more refined in their details.

Wedgewood pottery was popular during this period, with designs that mimicked Roman and Greek originals. One of the most striking differences from buildings of the older Georgian style is the use of both oval and octagonal room shapes in conjunction with elegant, elliptical staircases.

Another loose interpretation of classical Georgian/Adams style in ornamentation, although the hipped roofline is typical of later Greek Revival styles.

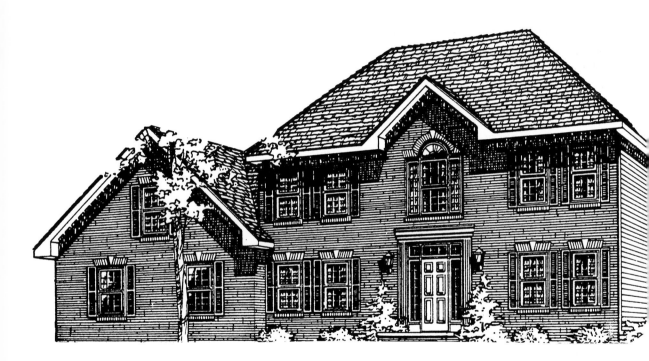

Greek Revival 1825 - 1850

Most often associated with Southern plantation mansions, Greek Revival houses had the neoclassical elements of Adams houses, with a shift toward greater opulence. These two- to three-story homes featured a low-pitched gabled or hipped roof. The porch varied from a simple, one-story entry to full height and width façades, while wide-banded cornices at the roof and porch were often evident.

The popularity of classical Greek architecture may be partially attributed to the political climate of the times, with the majestic elements of style seeming to embody the democratic ideals of a new and growing nation.

The bold and dignified appearance of this style caused it to be a common choice for public and governmental buildings. Pioneers heading westward along the Missouri River were deeply impressed with the grandeur of these structures. Upon settling in the new frontier, they would often temporarily erect a log cabin, which they would soon replace with a more permanent Greek Revival-inspired homestead.

The style was at its most charming when used on smaller, modestly scaled houses, and it remained popular into the turn of the century in the western states. In urban settings such as New York City, where it was especially in vogue, Greek Revival architecture took the form of brick and stone row houses with monumental, free-standing columns. Greek style architectural detailing was most often applied as porch columns; door and window surrounds; bold, wooden cornices with detailing of acanthus leaves; Greek key motifs; and other designs derived from the ancients. Major archaeological discoveries during this time period further fueled the enthusiasm for classical Greece.

Inside, elaborate plaster cornices and moldings topped plain plastered walls with 12-foot or even 14-foot ceilings. Set off by Ionic columns, pilasters and doorcases, walls were painted in soft pastel colors, tones of white, very light grays or light straw to complement the white painted woodwork.

Mantelpieces were bold yet simple, often constructed of beautifully figured black marble that was veined with gold. Furniture was fashioned of mahogany and rosewood, arranged in suites of matching pieces.

The use of wallpaper was common, with French scenic patterns in large scale being considered very chic. Fabrics of Chinese silk, velvets, damasks and woven tapestries would complete the look.

An imposing temple entry and heavy cornice trim show
Greek Revival influence in this contemporary interpretation.

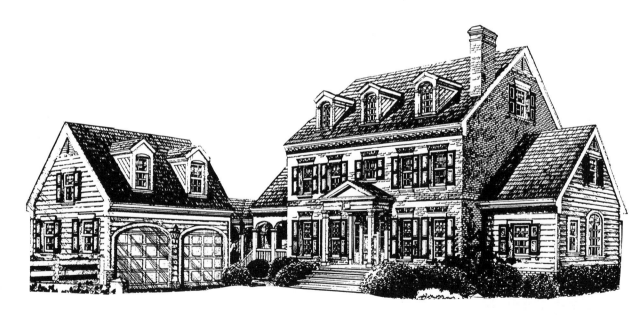

Typical Greek Revival with temple ends, corner pilasters and temple entrance.

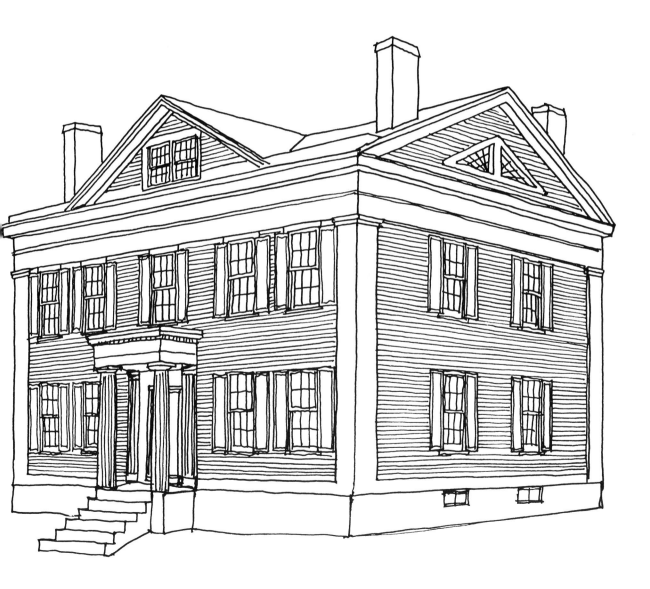

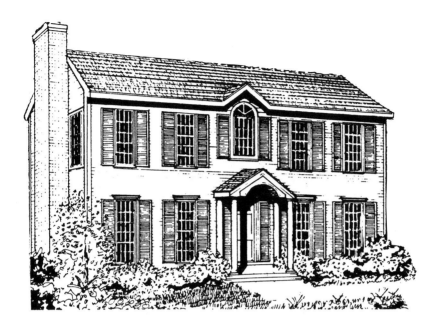

*A modified temple entry, repeated in the front
gable over a Palladian window, indicates Greek
Revival influence. Also, floor-to-ceiling
windows were a popular feature of this style.*

Greek Revival style was easily adaptable to popular use by the
middle classes, and carpenters and other craftspeople replicated the
elements of style freely. In fact, it is not uncommon to detect Greek
Revival elements on a simple Victorian farmhouse, or an early 20th
century bungalow.

Once detected and identified, a theme can be derived and carried
through into the home's interior, giving newfound dignity and
identity to an otherwise unremarkable structure.

Gothic Revival 1830 - 1875

The Gothic style was characterized by a steep-pitched roof with cross gables. Doors and windows had a pointed arch shape, often with decorative crowns. Lacy, jigsaw trim was found around the eaves and porches.

Gothic Revival example with trellis work at gable ends, steep-pitched roof and a mixture of siding materials.

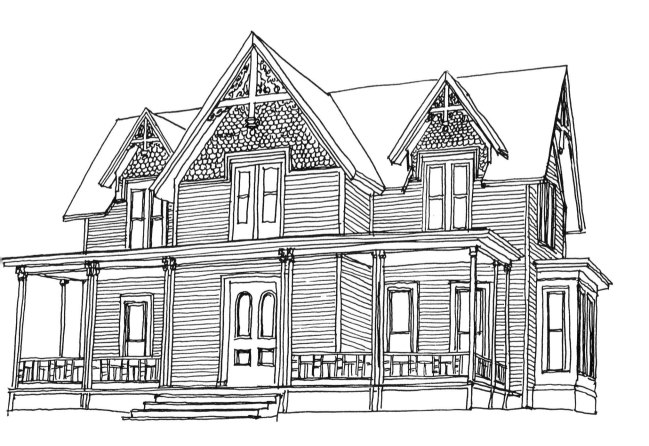

Appropriate for a small country cottage or a rambling villa of irregular plan and profile, this romantic style evoked a pastoral idealism. Andrew Jackson Downing, a horticulturist and philosopher of the mid 1800s, popularized this style in his books, and advised that homes be situated to take advantage of vistas in naturalistic and less formalized settings.

Much Gothic design originated in England, especially in ecclesiastic architecture, but Americans were more often inspired by romantic, sentimental notions of the past, with strong revivalist feelings often associated with the Medieval period. Gothic Revival elements were most commonly found adorning an otherwise Victorian structure, but the romantic notion of medieval, pastoral villages peopled with craft guilds struck a popular chord that offered an alternative to the social ills of the Industrial Age. In the Gothic Revival, we find the roots of the Arts and Crafts Movement of the early 20th century.

Example of Gothic Revival contemporary interpretation.

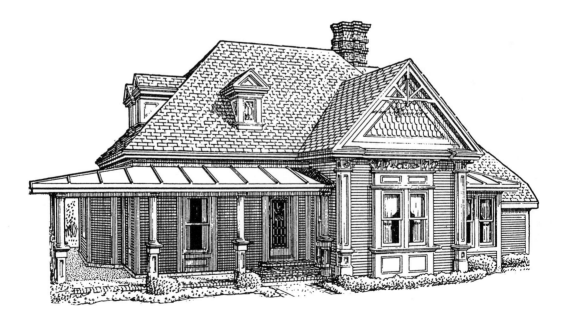

Gothic Revival interiors were characterized by dark oak or native wood beams and vaulted ceilings, frequently papered or painted with designs. Dominant doorways and massive fireplaces would lend a baronial air, while elaborate "linenfold" paneling, which resembles softly pleated fabric, would lend an elegant touch.

Trelliswork repeated from the exterior gables was used to adorn archways and windows, and diamond-paned, leaded glass windows were typical. Fabrics would consist of linens, velvets and tapestries, which would play off the rough-textured plaster walls painted in off-whites or soft, color-washed tints. Rich, jewel-tone colors with gilt accents, natural stone and wrought iron completed the scheme.

This example of design for new construction illustrates the rambling character that is noteworthy of Gothic Revival and its strong ties to Victorian styles.

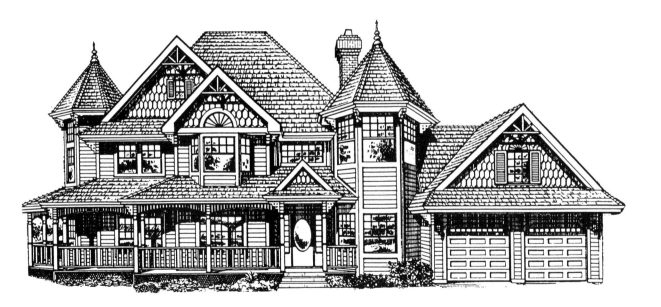

Victorians 1860 - 1900

Victorian architecture loosely parallels the reign of Queen Victoria, and comprises a vast diversity of styles and characters. The Industrial Age and the rapid growth of the railroads across America were important influences as well, leading to dramatic changes in the way homes were designed and built.

Balloon stick framing was introduced, providing a quicker, more economical and flexible way of construction, compared with the heavy timber framing technique that had been the standard since medieval times. No longer confined to box-like structures, flexible stick-framed houses could be built that incorporated wall extensions, overhangs and irregular ground plans.

Now, factories could pre-fabricate complex components, such as doors, windows, roofing, siding and decorative features, at relatively low costs. These could then be shipped via the railway network to building sites around the nation. Most Victorian styles are based on medieval prototypes, but little attempt was made to recreate the precise historical detailing.

The various Victorian styles tended to overlap each other, in contrast to the more clear-cut period styles that preceded them. Multi-textured, asymmetrical facades and steeply pitched roofs were common, but the period can be better identified and defined by dividing it into sub-groups.

Second Empire 1860 -1880

Napoleon III, nephew of Napoleon Bonaparte I, was making a name for himself and for France by, among other things, transforming the Paris of old into the city of grand boulevards that is known today. Following the example of his famous uncle, Napoleon III managed to have himself declared emperor, rather than being limited to a single-term presidency. He also set the fashion for a new style, dubbed the Second Empire.

The single most identifying feature of a Second Empire Victorian is its mansard roof. Named after 17th century French architect François Mansart, this unique roof profile allowed for an entire usable floor at the attic level, which, at the time it was originally developed, provided an additional rental floor in Parisian tenements where zoning ordinances limited the number of stories.

Second Empire with typical mansard roof profile.

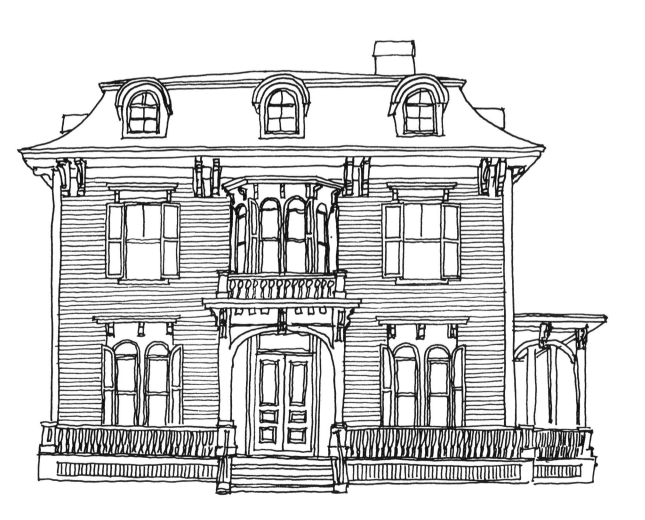

For this reason, in America, the style became a popular choice for the remodeling of earlier buildings. The roof is a double-pitched hip form with large dormer windows on the steep slope. The eaves are typically defined with heavy moldings and supported by brackets. Square cupolas and towers often accented the structures, with a roof line that was sometimes different from that of the main house.

Stick Victorian resplendent with decorative half-timbering and brackets.

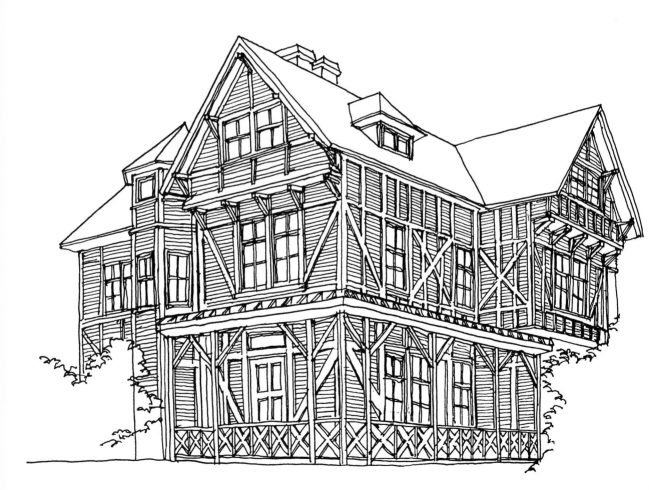

Stick Victorian 1860 -1890

Named by professor and architect Vincent Scully in the 1960s, this style originated from Victorians seeking to free themselves from European influences, while creating a new style that got its character from complexity of form and inventive expression of structure. Stick Victorian was a transitional style, linking Gothic Revival to the subsequent Queen Anne Victorian, which was to become far more influential and widespread.

Many Stick Victorian townhouses still survive, and can be found in San Francisco, where rapid growth and the abundance of lumber promoted the popularity of the style. Steeply pitched roofs, flamboyant projections, brackets and rafter tails combine with the principal feature of the Stick Victorian style: decorative stickwork trusses at the gables and shingle or board siding, interrupted by patterns of horizontal, vertical and diagonal boards that mimic the exposed structural half-timbering of medieval houses. It may be noted that the applied decoration had no structural relation to the underlying balloon frame construction.

The popularity of the Stick style grew as decorative elements were published in pattern books of the 1860s and 1870s. Vertical boards trimmed the sides of windows and the corners, which extended up into brackets at the eaves. Bay windows were usually box-like projections, often with sunburst motifs in gables and Eastlake trim above the windows and doors, mimicking the popular furniture style.

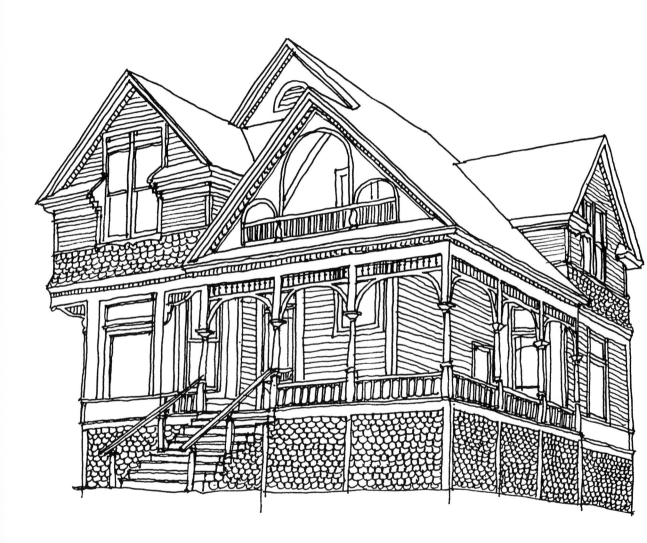

Queen Anne 1880 -1910

A group of 19th century architects named and popularized this style, which had little to do with the formal renaissance architecture that was typical of the reign of Queen Anne (1702-1714). Rather, the style borrows heavily from late medieval Elizabethan and Jacobean styles. Quasi-medieval, half-timbering patterned masonry is lifted from Tudor Revival styles, with spindlework and gingerbread trim among the more local adaptations.

The homes typically featured assertive chimneys, and were most often characterized by their varied surface patterning. Even if the house is completely sided in brick or in shingles, the alternating patterns would provide a variation of texture. The components for Queen Anne Victorians were often sold pre-cut by mail order companies. Knee-braces, brackets, spindles and other characteristic trim were also sold separately, and were used to embellish less decorative, pre-existing homes.

Porches and verandas flourished on Queen Anne Victorians, while turrets, towers and fanciful gazebos graced the more lavish examples of this style. Queen Anne homes were promoted to the nation in the first architectural magazine published in the United States, *The American Architect and Building News*. Because of the popularity of the style, Queen Anne houses of modest size often boasted architectural features such as towers, bays, porches and complicated woodwork.

Victorians are characterized by richly textured interiors and exteriors, which create a sense of visual complexity. Queen Anne homes display a more relaxed, informal air, with cozy interiors and a more comfortable, worn look. Lighter than "High Victorians," with their abundant draperies and eclectic interiors, the interiors of the Queen Anne Victorians were more in harmony with the incipient Arts and

← *Queen Anne example with wrap-around porch and informal, rambling style.*

Crafts movement. Many similar materials are appropriate, i.e., shingled siding and open floor plans. Major first-floor rooms usually opened onto the main living hall, from which an elegant main staircase rose ceremoniously to the second floor.

Victorian homes were frequently awash in wallpapered surfaces. Anaglypta and Lincrusta, heavily embossed and textured papers that were designed to be painted or glazed, were also popular, as was stamped tin, which was most commonly used on ceilings.

Modern-day Queen Anne, identified by its turret, porch and mix of siding materials.

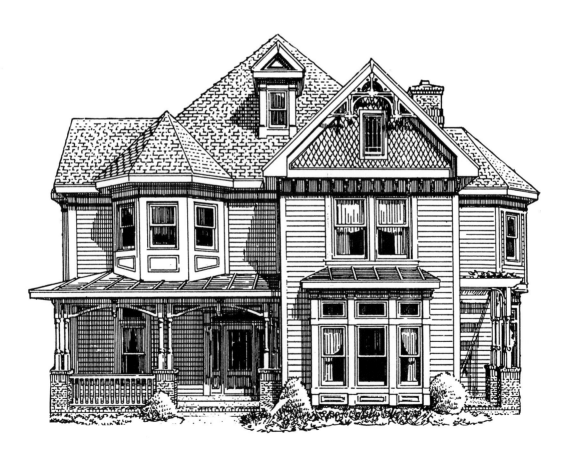

A more elaborate, modern Queen Anne with wrap-around porch, turret and fanciful turnposts at porch and railings.

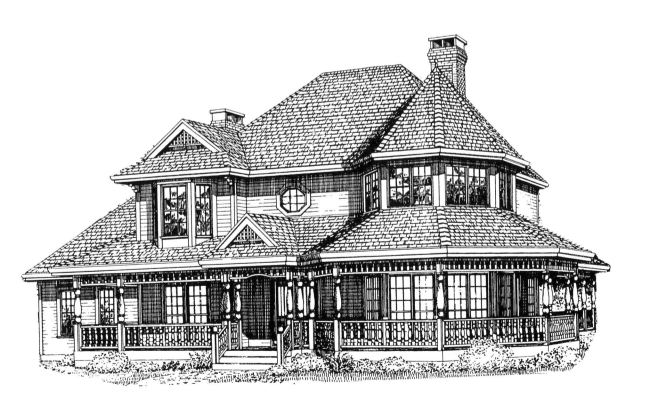

Shingle-style Victorians are easily identifiable by the use of shingle-siding that unifies projections, bays and porches into the mass of the house. Applied ornamentation is eliminated to emphasize the smooth flowing line of this style.

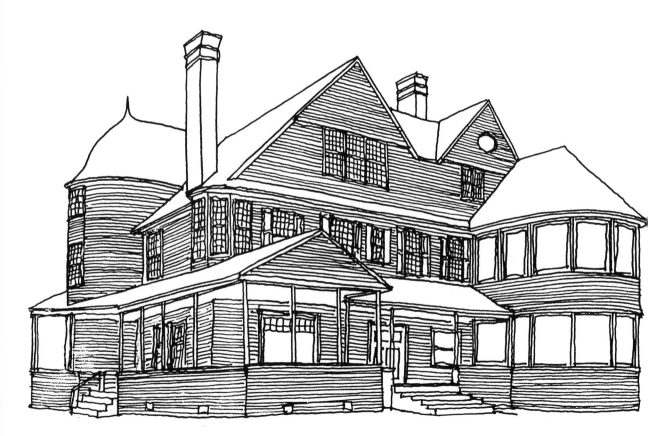

Shingle Style 1880 - 1900

Shingle style was a uniquely American adaptation and, as with the Queen Anne style, was primarily developed by architects. Wrap-around shingled exterior walls without cornerboards distinguished this style. Although the typical, asymmetrical Victorian façades were still present, decorative detailing at doors, windows, cornices and porches disappeared.

Extensive porches were still popular, as were steeply pitched roof lines with multi-level eaves. This time, however, the complex shapes were enclosed within a smooth, cohesive surface, with decorative detailing used only very sparingly. Towers closely resembled pronounced bays or half-towers, with roofs that blended into the main volume of the house. Bay windows, multiple windows and walls curving into windows were all common features of this style.

Decorative touches such as Palladian windows and simple classical columns were also borrowed from the emerging Colonial Revival styles. The Shingle Victorian reached its highest expression in seaside resorts designed by architects in the Northeastern states.

In general, the Victorians were associated with eclectic interiors which utilized intricate patterns and rich colors on carpets, walls and curtains. Displayed collections, such as shell boxes, silverware, porcelains and travel souvenirs, were also popular.

Fabrics patterned with tartans, heraldic emblems and lace were set off by floral wallpapers, creating a riot of color, pattern and rich texture. Many Victorian homes also gave evidence of the owner's fascination with travel, featuring an abundance of books, maps and globes.

Heavy mahogany, walnut or blackened oak furniture pieces would be combined with wicker and papier mâché pieces. The use of marble and tile became popular, especially in kitchens and bathrooms, where this material was favored for its ability to be kept "sanitary." Wood floors were polished frequently, and then covered with rich Oriental carpets.

A modern interpretation of the shingle style.

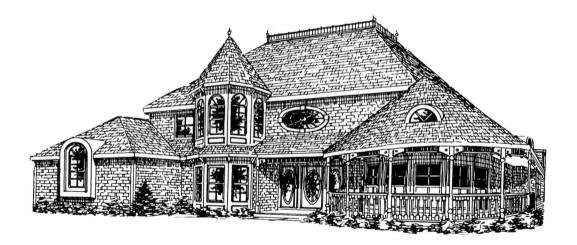

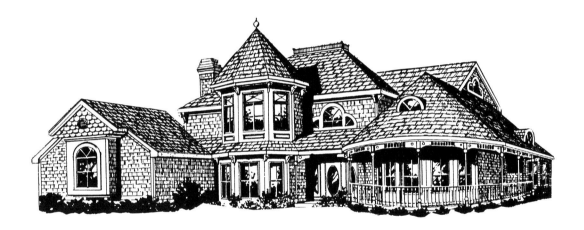

Victorian house with a contemporary look.

Folk and Vernacular Victorian
1870 - 1910

Folk and Vernacular are terms used to describe modest homes of the era. The growth of railroads and the popularity of builders' pattern books and catalogues made mass-produced, pre-cut detailing available to everyone from distant mills.

Many builders purchased this newly available trim and added onto traditional Folk house forms that were familiar to the local carpenters. Others simply updated older folk homes by dressing them up with new Victorian porches or other decorative features.

After 1910, this style was replaced by the Bungalow and "kit" Colonial Revival and Tudor Revival homes. On these, the façade was usually symmetrical and fairly simple, with lace-like spindles or flat jig-sawed "gingerbread" trim adorning the porches.

Sometimes Vernacular is a catch-all term used to describe any old house that doesn't have a readily identifiable style. These structures were most influenced by the use of materials that were locally available, as well as building techniques and skills available to local builders. Regional characteristics, such as climate, topography and availability of materials, are important to consider, if one is to understand what is Vernacular. For example, in New England, wood, brick, stone and steep-sloped roofs that would shed the snow are typical. In the Southwest, adobe, mud-brick and flat roofs dominated the earliest building styles. In the Midwest and Prairie states, logs, mud and thatch, as well as stone, were commonly used as building materials.

With the advent of the railroad and increased availability of prefabricated ornamental trims, even a modest regional structure could be "dressed up" with some fancy Victorian trimwork, resulting in some very interesting and unusual combinations. Not surprisingly, Vernacular styles were most commonly found in farmhouses and smaller rural homes; however, it is not uncommon to find a pocket neighborhood of Vernacular Victorians in an urban setting, especially in an old "working class" district.

Folk Vernacular Victorians often incorporated factory-made ornamentation that was added to an earlier Colonial structure for a more stylish look.

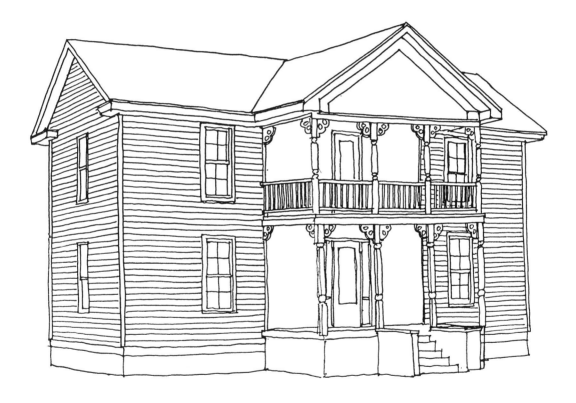

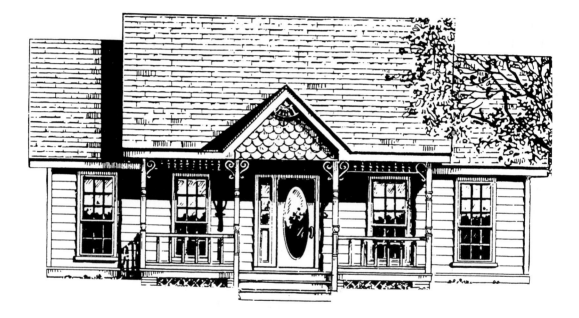

*This modest modern Victorian could be described as
Vernacular with its gingerbread trim and turnposts at
porch and entry adorning an otherwise simple structure.*

Picturesque
1890 - 1930

These opulent housing styles, which included Romanesque, Chateauesque, Beaux Arts, Grand Tudor, Italian Renaissance Revival and Neoclassical Revival, grew up more or less concurrently with the Victorian and subsequent Colonial Revival periods. These were the mansions of America's super-rich, "The Four Hundred," as they were dubbed at the time.

In 1892, the Census Bureau estimated that nine percent of the nation's families owned 71 percent of the wealth. The fantastic growth of industry and the railroads created an elite class of super rich who were transforming rural farmlands into palatial estates, thanks to the commuter railways that enabled them to commute into the cities and tend to their business interests.

Enjoying the power and comfort of their newfound wealth, these families sought to establish their positions in society through membership in exclusive clubs, philanthropic organizations and foundations.

The first *Social Register* was published in 1887, and the American aristocracy was in full swing. With the aristocracy complaining that the Shingle Style Victorians and Colonial Revivals were not ostentatious enough, architects were pressed into service to create more impressive and palatial homes, such as the Vanderbilt's "Baltimore" estate (Chateauesque), built in North Carolina in 1893 at an estimated cost in excess of $6 million.

Other landmarks, such as The Breakers (Beaux Arts), in Newport, Rhode Island; the Weringen House (Grand Tudor), in Cleveland, Ohio; and the Phelan House (Italian Renaissance Revival), in Saratoga, California, seemed to rival the royal castles of Europe. Noteworthy architectural firms that catered to immensely wealthy clients included Richard Morris Hunt; McKim, Mead & White; and Warren & Westmore.

While it is unlikely that kitchen and bathroom designers will be called upon frequently to work on surviving examples from this period, further study of these styles is encouraged, as it can serve as a springboard of ideas and inspiration in design work. Furthermore, many of the architectural details can be adapted and incorporated into our theme designs of today. It is fortunate that many of these palatial structures are public buildings or historic landmarks that we can continue to study, tour and learn from, even today.

A Chateauesque mansion from the opulent era of the Picturesque styles. →

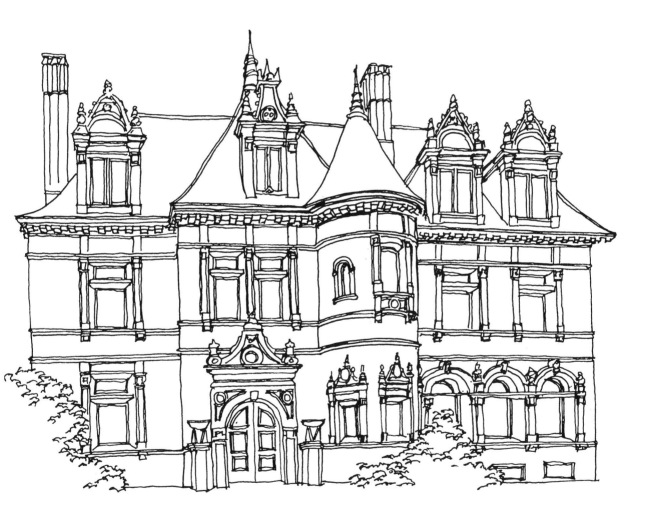

Craftsman 1890 - 1930

More than an architectural style, the Arts and Crafts movement was a philosophy that influenced and fostered a whole new way of life. Its roots date back to England in the mid-1800s, to a group of Medieval Revivalists who longed for the simpler, more wholesome days of 17th century "merrie olde England."

A typical Craftsman-style bungalow from the early part of the 20th century.

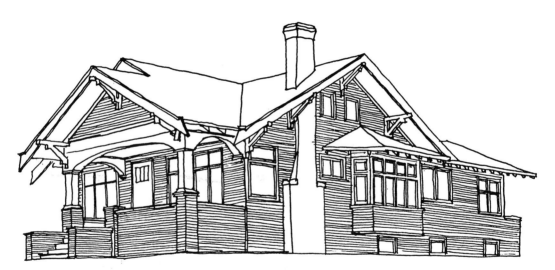

In fact, England in the mid-1800s was rampant with a general, deep-rooted sense of dissatisfaction, the result of the Industrial Revolution, with its unfortunate by-products of pollution and exploitation of the working class, including children. The products that were mass produced at this time were often of shoddy, poor quality.

William Morris and his mentor, John Ruskin, led a group of intellectuals and architects who romanticized the medieval crafts guilds, where the craftsmen produced honestly designed, well-executed products in an atmosphere that was conducive to the simple life. Their traditional, English Country cottages were considered to be the inspiration for the Craftsman style.

Arts and Crafts architects followed the general rules of the country builder, stressing common sense and practicality in their designs, which used local materials and building techniques. In their hands, the humble country cottage became conscious architecture.

The idea that well-designed goods of every kind should be made available to all levels of society was one that would ultimately reform the tastes of the middle class. However, in England and throughout Europe, the movement met with limited success, as the cost of high-quality handcrafted goods continued to make them inaccessible to the common person.

In Europe, the movement evolved more or less into Art Nouveau, under the guidance of such inventive leaders as the architect, Charles Rennie Macintosh. William Morris and his cronies were generally recognized as extreme Socialists and a little too much out of the mainstream for conservative English sensibilities.

In America, the father of the Arts and Crafts movement was Gustav Stickley, a simple furniture maker who was not an architect, an aristocrat or an intellectual. He ultimately ended up designing houses to accommodate his furniture. Stickley reacted with distaste to the contemporary trend of mass production, coupled with declining quality. He believed that the highly ornate, High Victorian curlicues and fretwork added nothing of value to his furniture.

Thus, he carried out the Craftsman theme from finely crafted, simple and sturdy furniture to textiles, pottery and, eventually, house designs.

Stickley also published *The Craftsman Magazine*, which included plans for furniture and houses, as well as articles on the benefits of the Craftsman lifestyle. He provided detailed house plans free of charge to subscribers of his magazine, and urged home builders to modify and personalize these plans to suit individual needs, climate, availability of local materials, and the builder's abilities and expertise. For this reason, it is impossible to say how many Craftsman homes were actually built during this period.

Modern-day bungalow. Sidelights and clerestory windows over entry door were not typical.

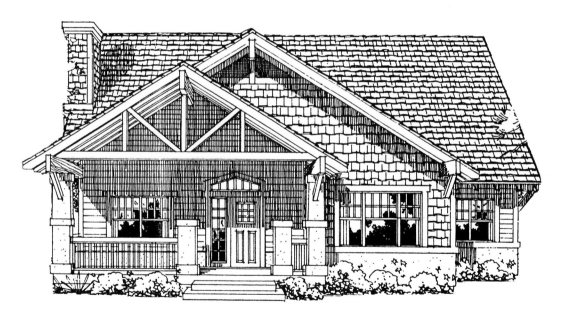

However, America's growth spurt between 1900 and the 1920s produced many cottages, bungalows and structures that were either pure Craftsman or Craftsman-inspired and adapted. The Craftsman style remained popular throughout the 1920s in vacation homes and modest suburbs throughout the country.

Sears and Roebuck, Aladdin Redi-Cut and other manufacturers of pre-cut "kit" houses shipped Craftsman-style houses wherever there were train tracks to carry them. The homes could even be ordered through mail-order catalogs. As a result, a flood of pattern books appeared, offering plans for Craftsman bungalows, making the one- to one-and-a-half-story Craftsman bungalow the most popular and fashionable smaller house in the country.

High style interpretations were executed by West Coast architectural firms of Greene and Greene, Bernard Maybeck and Julia Morgan. Frank Lloyd Wright, a later Arts and Crafts architect, used the style as a springboard for his unique Prairie style.

This style is generally identified by its low-pitched, gabled and sometimes hipped roof line, with wide eave overhangs. Roof rafters are usually exposed, with decorative false beams or braces added under the gables. Also typical of this style are dominant porches with their roofs supported by tapered, square columns or pedestals which frequently extended to the ground.

Craftsman houses are characterized by the rustic texture of the building materials, and are often embellished with extensive pergolas and trellises, lending a distinctive Oriental flavor to the style. The color and tone of the houses were usually derived from natural materials such as brick, stone or shingles with an earth-toned stain applied to them.

Craftsman doors and windows are similar to those used in Prairie style houses. Dormers are commonly gabled or shed, with exposed rafter ends and braces similar to those used in the main roof wall junctions. Secondary influences such as Tudor false half-timbering, Swiss balustrades or Oriental up-turned roof forms are sometimes incorporated as well.

A wonderfully accurate and well-detailed modern interpretation of the classic Craftsman style.

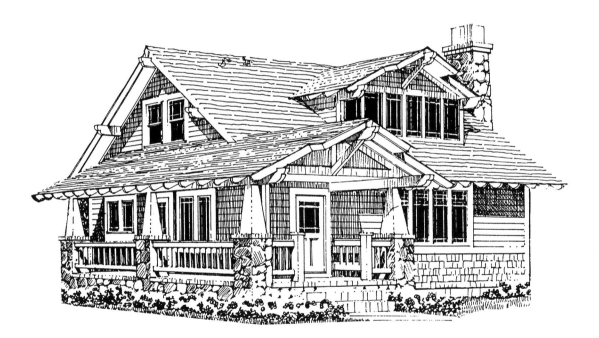

Craftsman style homes were intended to be comfortable, natural in appearance and, if possible, appointed with well-crafted handmade objects. Furniture was typically constructed of fumed white oak, embellished only by the fine grain of the wood and the craftsmanship of the joinery. Wicker furniture was used to alleviate the heaviness of the solid wood pieces. Softly colored fabrics of textured natural linen, flax and woven tapestries added to the interior ambiance.

Muddy earth colors, mossy greens, ochre-yellows, grayish blues and natural wood tones were considered compatible with natural surroundings, and helped to link the interior with the outdoors.

The use of comfortable, durable, easy-care furnishing and accessories was also encouraged, which carried over into the design of kitchens and bathrooms in Craftsman homes.

Other typical interior elements include partially paneled walls (to about 5 feet in height), often topped by a book or plate shelf supported by chunky brackets; tile fronted fireplaces, sometimes fitted with copper hoods; inglenook seating around the hearth; and broad, cased openings between rooms.

Prairie 1900 - 1920

Architect Frank Lloyd Wright built a Shingle Victorian for his family in Oak Park, Illinois, before he developed his famous regional Prairie style. Influenced by the principles of the Arts and Crafts Movement, he took the Bungalow style to more sophisticated and refined heights. Joined by a creative group of Chicago architects now known as the Prairie School, Wright has been widely acknowledged as master of the Prairie style house.

Prairie style homes were usually two stories high, sometimes with a single-story outstretched wing. Low-pitched, hipped roofs with wide overhanging eaves are also typical of this style. Bands of casement windows, often with abstract, geometric patterns of stained glass, established a strong horizontal emphasis. Also commonly featured were massive, square porch supports, window boxes or flattened pedestal urns for flowers, broad flat chimneys, porte chocheres and covered porches extending out from the main core of the house.

Horizontal bands of windows and low-hipped rooflines with wide overhangs are the most recognizable elements of this type, pioneered by Frank Lloyd Wright and his Chicago-area associates.

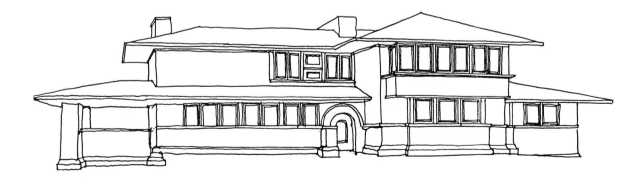

Prairie houses were built to act in harmony with the regional landscape, and, in fact, the Prairie School tended to reject details derived from traditional European traditions, instead developing new decorative motifs.

The Prairie style originated in Chicago and was fostered in and around other large, Midwestern cities. Vernacular examples could be found in pattern books and popular magazines. It is widely believed that the Prairie style evolved (or degenerated, depending on how you view it) into the post World War II ranch-style houses that crowd our suburbs today.

A contemporary interpretation of Prairie style, this house incorporates the low-pitched hipped rooflines with wide overhangs and horizontal detail, but the vertical composition of the windows is a departure.

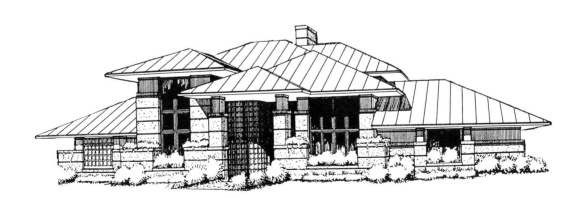

Colonial Revival 1885 - 1955

The Colonial Revival style grew popular as a result of a reawakening of pride in America's colonial past, following the nation's centennial celebration of 1876. This style also offered a refreshing alternative to the excesses of Victorian architecture.

Colonial styles were loosely adapted from early English and Dutch houses of the Atlantic seaboard. Georgian and Adams styles were the most predominant, with secondary influences coming from medieval English and Dutch Colonial prototypes.

Although Georgian Palladian windows were used extensively, they were generally larger and grouped in pairs. Colonial Revival windows were also larger than their originals, usually with divided lights on the upper sashes. They, too, were used in pairs, unlike the original prototypes from which they were derived.

Early Colonial Revival houses employed 18th century details and applied them to simplified Queen Anne and Shingle housing forms. Unfortunately, there was a lot of free association, and proportions and scale were not always accurately reproduced. Generally speaking, the houses were much larger than the original Colonials. Later in the life of this prolific style, details were more carefully researched and duplicated.

The Dutch Colonials, a major subgroup of the Colonial Revivals, were characterized by their gambrel roof, where one or both of the lower roof slopes flares at the eaves, suggesting a gentle curve. Most examples are one story high, with a steeply pitched gambrel roof that contains almost a full second story, reminiscent of the Second Empire Victorian style. The Dutch Colonials use either separate dormers or a continuous shed dormer with several windows.

Side, flat-roofed porches or sunrooms are typical in both Colonial Revivals and Dutch Colonials. The front door is emphasized with moldings, decorative crown or pediment supported by pilasters.

Doors commonly utilize either fanlights above or sidelights. The typical Colonial Revival façade is symmetrical, with paired windows of multi-pane glazing.

The Classic Box, or Foursquare, was another popular Colonial Revival style among the working class. Most of these were built before 1915, and featured a hipped roof with a full width porch at the

Colonial Revival style incorporates design elements from Georgian, Adams and Greek Revival styles.

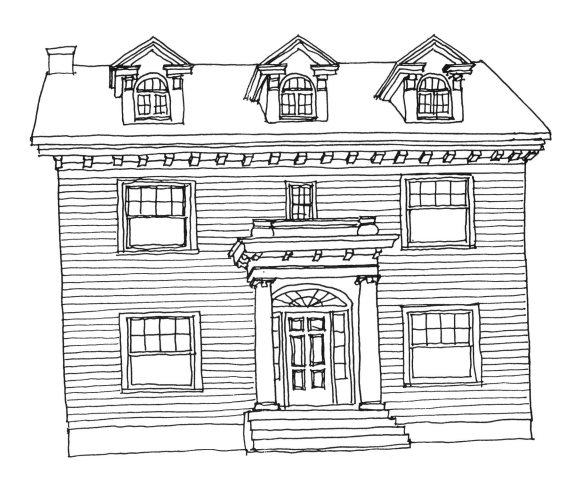

front, supported by classical columns. Square or rectangular in plan, they were sometimes embellished with full height pilasters at the corners, and symmetrically placed dormers, either hipped, gabled or shed-roofed. This style overlapped with the popularity of the Craftsman Bungalows, and shares many of the same clean, no-frills features.

A Palladian entry, Greek Revival porch and Georgian ornamentation grace this Colonial Revival classic.

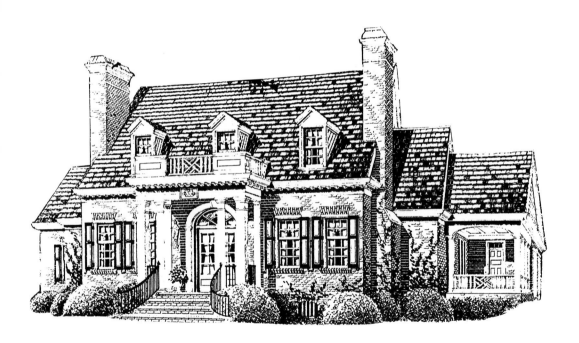

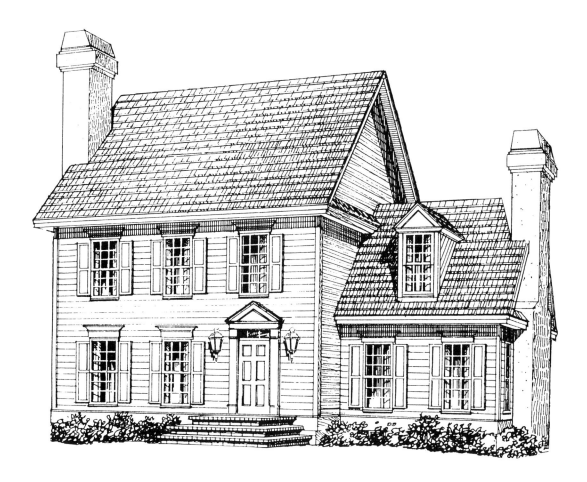

This Colonial Revival design follows Adams style detailing very closely.

Interiors were brightened with flowered chintz, often using the same pattern on wall coverings, upholstery and window treatments. Light woods were popular, but so was mahogany in Sheraton and Duncan Phyfe suites. Moldings and woodwork were painted white, and hardwood floors were covered with grand Oriental carpets, or perhaps tiled with black and white marble. Ornaments were confined to high shelves, as rooms were kept open and spacious, a conscious effort to break from Victorian clutter.

Repetitive use of classical elements, such as the Palladian arch in this case, is typical of the Colonial Revival style. The simplified, squared columns are an interpretation of the classical originals.

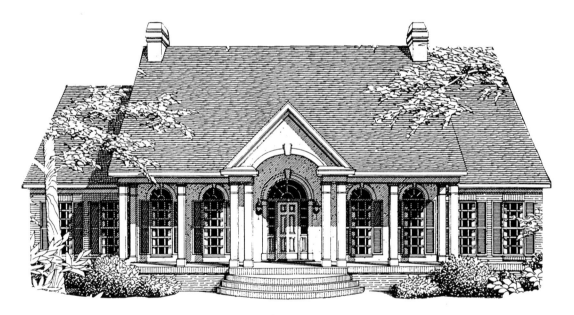

Tudor Revival 1900 - 1940

This style is loosely derived from medieval English examples, varying from thatched roof cottages to grand manor estates. It is characterized by a steeply pitched roof, often cross gabled, with decorative half timbering. Windows are typically tall and narrow, often with a transom or clerestory above. Leaded, diamond-paned windows were frequently used in the more important locations. Massive chimneys with a decorative finial or chimney pot at the top were commonly featured as well.

Tudor Revival was extremely popular in the early 1920s and 1930s. Accordingly, stucco, brick or stone cladding was typical, with wooden cladding less common.

A very decorative and romantic style, the Tudor Revival homes usually boasted interiors that carried out the theme set by its architecture. Principal rooms had an air of adventure and exploration. Walls were paneled, with built-in bookcases and cabinetry. Stone-faced or tiled fireplaces with a Tudor arch would adorn the living space, as would exposed wooden beams, wrought iron and leaded glass.

Heraldic motifs, heavy tapestries, leather and deep, jewel-tone colors would complete the environment. Then, as now, antiques and furnishings with distressed finishes were used to add the patina of age as well as a sense of established comfort and rich heritage.

Typical Tudor Revival style with decorative half timbering, diamond-paned windows and steep rooflines.

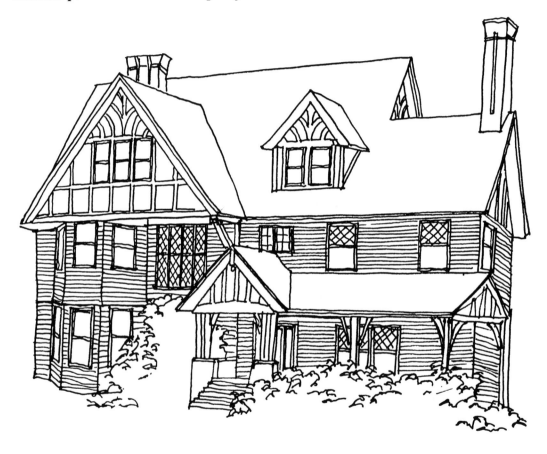

This Tudor Revival is a classic interpretation of the English country cottage.

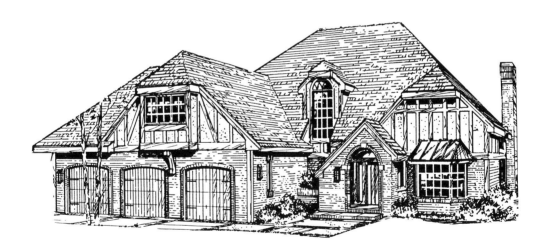

*Example of contemporary **Tudor Revival** style.*

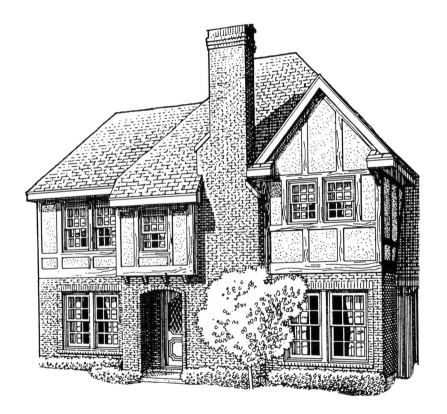

Spanish Mission and
Spanish Colonial 1910 - 1930

In the West and the Southwest, Colonial Revival meant looking back to the early Spanish styles for inspiration. Characterized by low-pitched, barrel or S-shaped tiled roofs and stucco walls incorporating arched windows and doors, the style uses decorative details borrowed from Moorish, Byzantine, Gothic and Mediterranean influences. Although the style was most popular in the Southwest, its influence was spread with the help of the Southern Pacific and Santa Fe Railroad, which used the style for its stations and resort hotels.

Early Spanish Mission styles often included towers, tile roofs and stucco siding.

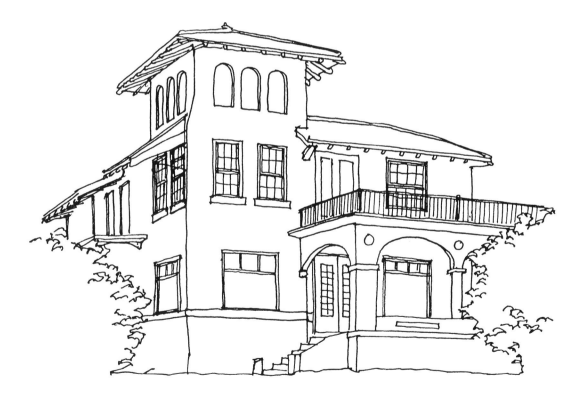

The true Spanish Mission style often incorporated an ornate parapeted gable end or central dormer, much like the early California missions built by the Spaniards. Spanish Colonials were more Mediterranean-influenced, often incorporating a central patio or court, which was popular in Florida as well as on the West Coast. Low-pitched tile roofs, stucco walls and heavy wooden doors with ornamental ironwork embellishing windows were common. The Spanish Colonial's characteristic U-shape, with a protected patio,

This modern Spanish Mission type combines grander Mediterranean influences with Early Mission style.

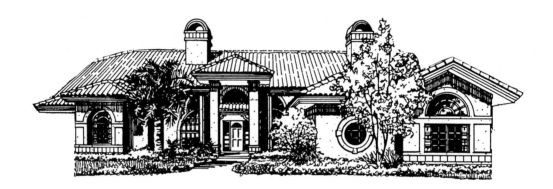

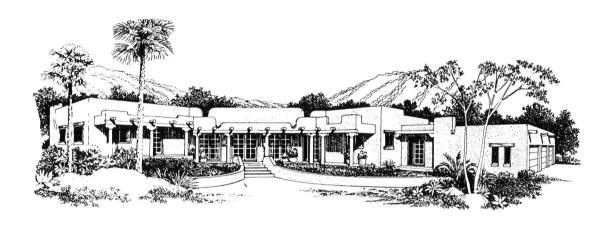

This Pueblo style is more typical of Southwestern United States' architecture.

was derived from the early Southwestern ranchos of the 19th century, and provided the basic formula for the ranch houses of today.

Many modestly scaled Spanish Mission and Spanish Colonial homes were modified Bungalows that were Spanish only in the appearance of their exteriors. Interior details were utilitarian with Spanish-style decor limited to wrought iron railings and tiled fireplaces.

Hardwood oak or tiled terra cotta floors were popular, and heavy plastered walls were painted in pastel colors, especially pink and peach. Craftsman "Mission" furniture was particularly appropriate, as were Baroque, Mediterranean and Gothic furnishings. Native American woven rugs, leather and patterned ceramics were used to enhance the environment.

Art Moderne 1920 - 1940

This style was an outgrowth of the earlier Art Deco style, which was typically used in public and commercial buildings in the early 1920s and 1930s. Art Deco was employed during that time as an interior design and fashion format, and was actually very rare in domestic architecture.

The Finnish architect Saarinen was a prominent Art Deco-influenced designer. Modernistic styling in buildings and houses came a little later, reflecting the streamlined styling popular in industrial design, such as trains, automobiles and ships. Curved lines, smooth surfaces and strong horizontal emphasis are major features of the style.

The strong horizontal emphasis links this style with earlier Prairie and Craftsman designs. However, Art Moderne structures have a more characteristic streamlined form, as if they would move through an airstream with no resistance. Roofs were typically flat, with parapet ledges, sometimes decorated in zigzag or chevron motifs. Glass block, small porthole windows, stucco, pipe railing, towers and other vertical projections were common, with decorative detailing kept to a minimum.

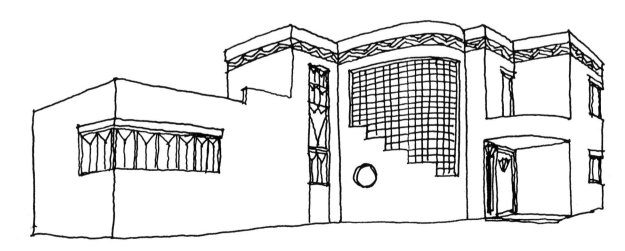

International 1930 - 1990

European architects, such as France's Le Corbusier and Germany's Mies Van der Rohe and Walter Gropius, pioneered this style in the years between World War I and World War II. While the predominant American styles were more traditional, the avant-garde group was busy re-defining architecture without historic precedent, using the materials and technology of the present.

Walls were not used for structural support, as in traditional architecture, but rather as curtains strung over a structural, usually steel, skeleton. Huge walls of glass were possible, with perhaps the most famous domestic example being Phillip Johnson's Glass House. Generally, preferences ran to smooth wall surfaces, stucco, smooth boards and sometimes brick or stone. Cantilevered projections for roofs, balconies or second stories were utilized to dramatize the non-supporting nature of the walls.

Classic International Style.

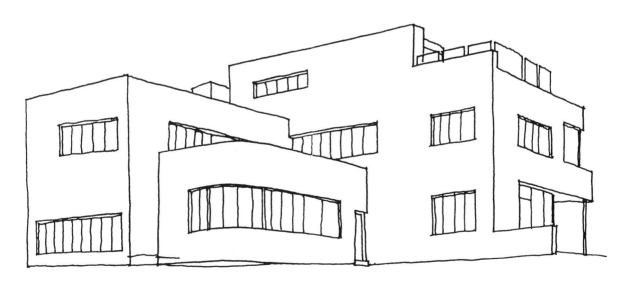

Le Corbusier promoted the idea of the house as a "machine for living," linking the architecture to the rapidly evolving technology of the times.

The Internationalists deplored decoration of any kind. Their kitchens and bathrooms would employ the latest technology and boast state-of-the-art functionalism, bringing true efficiency into the home. The International style also emphasized using form and structure to serve its inhabitants. Volume replaced mass as a major design consideration, and the exteriors of International style houses served only to shelter the inhabitants from the elements, and to express the nature of the inner structural core. Surfaces were usually painted or left pure white.

Contemporary interpretation of International style. The gabled roof and the low-brick trim would not be typical.

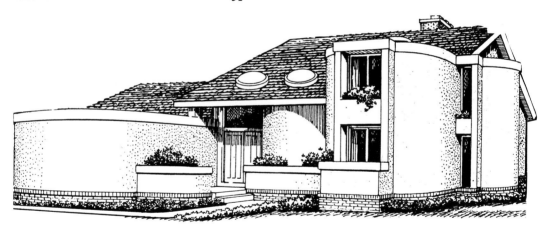

OVERLAY OF ARCHITECTURAL
STYLES, PERIODS AND INTERIOR THEMES

STYLE	PERIOD	THEME
English and Dutch Colonials	1650 - 1750	Colonial Shaker Swedish Country English Country
Georgian and Adams	1730 - 1820	Georgian Adams Neoclassical English Country French Country
Greek Revival	1825 - 1850	Neoclassical Biedermeier Federal and Empire
Gothic Revival	1830 - 1875	Tudor Jacobean English Country Baroque
Victorian	1860 - 1900	Regency Second Empire Baroque
Second Empire		Regency Directoire Jacobean
Stick *Queen Anne*		Tudor French Country English Country Georgian Edwardian
Shingle		Edwardian Arts and Crafts English Country
Folk		American Country Farmhouse

STYLE	PERIOD	THEME
Picturesque	1890 - 1930	Edwardian Beaux Arts Italianette Italian Country Art Nouveau Tudor
Craftsman	1890 - 1930	Arts and Crafts Tudor Lodge Style
Prairie	1900 - 1920	Arts and Crafts Prairie Contemporary Art Deco
Colonial Revival	1885 - 1955	Early Colonial Georgian Adams Queen Anne English Country
Tudor Revival	1900 - 1940	Tudor Jacobean Baroque Medieval Rustic
Spanish Revival	1910 - 1930	Arts and Crafts Italian Country Southwestern Tudor
Moderne	1920 - 1940	Art Nouveau Art Deco Savoy Biedermeier
International	1930 - 1990	Bauhaus Contemporary

PART II
THEME STYLES FOR KITCHENS AND BATHROOMS

Interior Styles and How To Use Them

With the foundation of knowledge and reference covered in the first part of this book, kitchen and bathroom design professionals can incorporate this information and develop the skills to "read" the houses they may have occasion to work on. There may be only very subtle clues in the applied ornamentation and the actual massing of a house that can allow us to determine how to add appropriately, in keeping with the integrity of the structure, or give us the confidence to remove inappropriate ornamentation to restore original style to a house with dramatic success. Eliminating shutters where they don't belong, or removing some Colonial Revival trim from a Vernacular Victorian or a stately Bungalow can be just the trick to give a sense of presence to an otherwise unremarkable home. Driving through a neighborhood and learning to pick out elements that don't belong can provide a diverting intellectual stimulation, but more practically, enhancing your knowledge of architectural styles gives you the foundation to build your theme designs in the kitchens and bathrooms within the walls. When you can recognize a house's style or even its suggested style, as in new construction, you can start a logical process in designing the interior spaces.

One of the first steps in planning for a kitchen or bathroom remodel is analyzing the space to determine if the client's stated needs can be met within the existing space. With a clear sense of the house's style, the form a proposed addition will take will be determined by how it will affect the main structure, and how it will fit in with the style of the house. Even the selection of windows and doors should be governed by how they will blend with the existing rhythm that has already been established. The most successful additions do not look as if they have been added on, which is the constant challenge of the professional remodeler. Our additions and remodelings may be so extensive that they actually create the style for the house, and require us to be very skillful designers, indeed.

The theme styles are outlined here to provide you with a handy reference. They are organized more or less chronologically, and whenever possible, are actually linked with the historic architectural style with which they would be most compatible. These are more guidelines than hard and fast rules, as there will be the inevitable exceptions. For example, a dramatic Gothic interior in an International-style modernistic home could be accomplished with spectacular success, as unlikely as it sounds. Most importantly, the style outlines are not intended to curb your creative impulses with strict rules, but to provide you with basic tools with which you can blend your clients' tastes and lifestyles with a flair of professional, skillful and, hopefully, timeless design that will serve them for years to come, and provide you with happy clients and future referrals.

Theme Styling Terminology

After designers have studied the history of architecture and understand the homes of our country, specific periods of design and styles of furniture can be identified. These eras are commonly called period styles. To clarify terminology used:

- **Period**: a particular time in history.
- **Style**: the work of a specific designer, or design period.
- **Traditional**: designs that come from past generations.
- **Country**: how a style is detailed; however, here it is used to define an informal version of a style.
- **Modern**: a style which is associated with and fabricated from currently used materials.
- **Contemporary**: a look which reflects the lifestyle of the current society. The design combines styles from diverse periods.
- **Eclectic**: mixing elements of different styles.
- **Motif**: generally the overall decorative scheme of an interior. Specifically, a motif is a pattern, design, emblem or object which has become automatically associated with a particular style.
- **Vernacular**: locally adapted from a formal style, exhibiting notable ethnic and regional interpretations—usually in rural or provincial areas. Mixing of traditions and new adaptations and ideas is common.

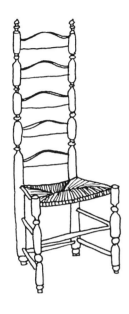

Early American ladder-back chair with woven rush seat.

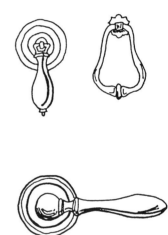

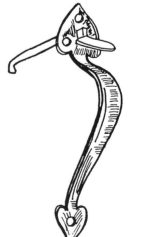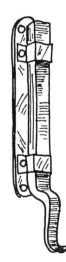

Typical early Colonial hardware would be crafted out of wrought iron, dull pewter or, less commonly, burnished, dull brass.

EARLY AMERICAN
Early Colonial

Historic Context
The Early Colonial styles find their roots in Early American themes. Rustic, medieval-style building techniques kept details simple and spare. Early Colonial interiors were warm and richly textured, with a rough and unsophisticated edge to them. The typical Colonial home combined rustic, handmade furnishings with a rare, occasional grand piece that would be the centerpiece of the room. The early Puritans were proud of their homes and their possessions which were openly displayed when possible or practical. Early Colonial kitchens were crowded rooms, usually the hub of daily activities, as well as gathering spots in the evening hours and at mealtimes.

Walls/Ceilings
Plastered or paneled walls have wide wood planks, with little molding detail. Wall colors are cool whites, peach, cream, apricots, subtle blues, greens and browns or slightly faded earthy reds. Stenciled border patterns are common.

Windows/Doors
Casement windows have small-paned glazing, simply trimmed, and doors would be wide, frame and flat panel or heavy planks. Split Dutch doors are also common.

Moldings
Light, small-scale molding strips at paneling would be used, and flat-board trims around windows, doors and at bases.

Cabinetry
Natural or darkened natural wood tones of pine, cherry, pecan, hickory or maple would be typical, with painted finishes in dull sheen "milk paints" of iodine reds, chalky subtle blues, mossy greens and browns. Distressed or dragged finishes give a worn, aged look. Unfitted styling with an occasional grand piece used as a focal point.

Countertops

Wood or wood-patterned, slate or ceramic tile are common. The feeling is rustic and textural.

Floors

Wide-planked and pegged wood floors in pine or oak would be used, as well as flagstone, slate or brick. Coverings might be woven cotton or braided rag rugs, sisal matting or Oriental rugs in faded tones.

Fabrics

These would include quilting, soft wools, homepsuns, linens patterned in checks, solids and damask patterns.

Designed by Alan Asnarow, CKD; Photos by John Schwartz

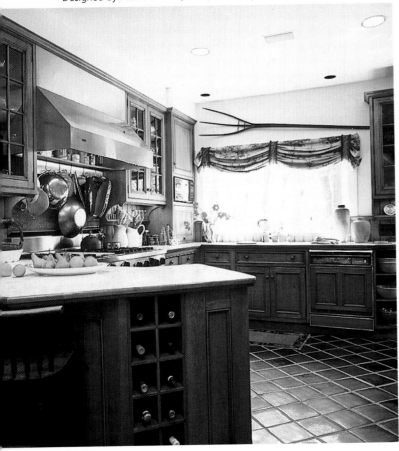

The distressed, aged finish on these pine cabinets and the stone floor is typical of Early Colonial style. The oversized commercial range and hood replace a large, open hearth. Crown molding is kept simple and minimal. Plank wainscoting and brick backsplash at range demonstrate effective use of appropriate materials to the style. Glass door cabinets with mullions mimic small-paned windows which would be found in Early Colonial homes.

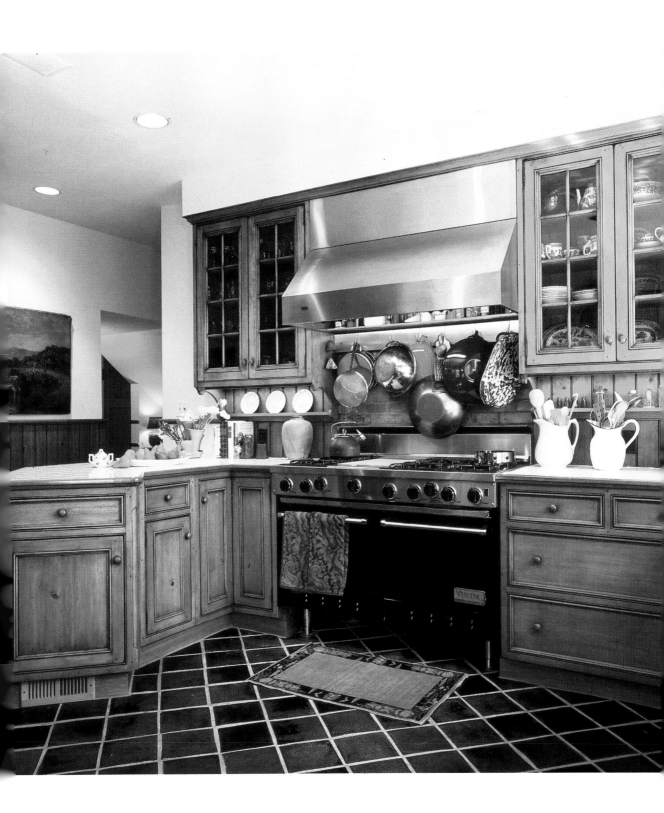

Wall Coverings

Small, primitive patterns or damask-type floral motifs would be appropriate, usually tone on tone or in pale colors on white or cream backgrounds—nothing too formal or grand.

Accessories

Pewter, silver, pottery pitchers, pots and slipware, wooden platters, bowls and baskets would be found.

This example of a Colonial kitchen illustrates the many activities that would typically take place in this busy room. Children, servants and the lady of the house populate the space.

Photo courtesy of Kathleen Donohue

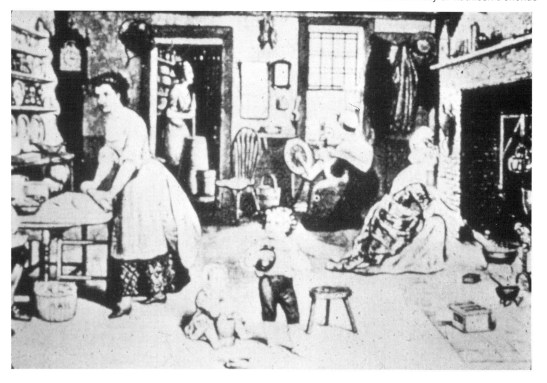

Stamped tin cabinet door inserts mimic Colonial pie safes. Metal tole-ware chandelier, colorful crockery and hanging cookware contribute to the Early Colonial theme. While the cherry wood of the cabinets is a little elegant for the style, its warmth and rich color readily blend into the theme. Ceramic knobs help to informalize the look.

Photo courtesy of NKBA

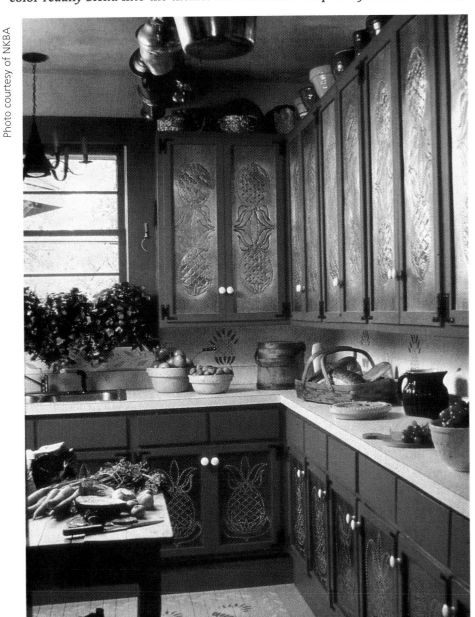

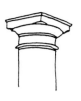

Doric-order capitals

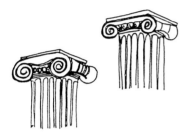

Ionic-order capitals   *Corinthian-order capitals*

*Georgian, Adams and Greek Revival styles
emphasized the use of the classical orders
of design elements from Roman and
Greek examples.*

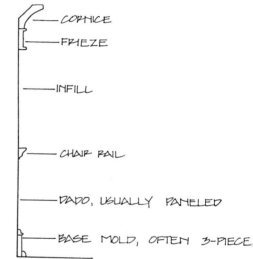

— CORNICE

— FRIEZE

— INFILL

— CHAIR RAIL

— DADO, USUALLY PANELED

— BASE MOLD, OFTEN 3-PIECE

*Typical classical compound molding systems derived from the capitals
and bases of Roman columns.*

COMPOUND CROWN   BASE MOLD

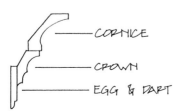

— CORNICE

— CROWN

— EGG & DART

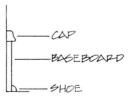

— CAP

— BASEBOARD

— SHOE

CLASSICAL
Georgian and Adams/Federal

Historic Context

Since Georgian and Adams styles make extensive use of the classical forms of Greek and Roman design, it's important to design the interior of the home in such a way that would place great emphasis on balance and symmetry. The first step to doing this would be to consider symmetrical placement of the windows, doors and openings.

Walls/Ceilings

Wall colors in rich, jewel tones help to highlight painted moldings. Ceilings might be barrel-vaulted and coffered.

Windows/Doors

Symmetrically placed, Palladian-style arched focal windows are typical, with 10-light French doors and solid raised panel doors.

Moldings

Very important would be grand friezes, cornices, pillars and pilasters. Classical designs such as dentil, egg and dart, Greek key, acanthus leaf, Vitruvian scroll and bay leaf garlands are incorporated. Compound crowns are built up from several moldings; base moldings are heavy. Use of molding and paneling are keynotes of this style. Often painted in glossy finishes, but rich wood tones like cherry, mahogany or walnut are also common. Faux-painted moldings are appropriate, with some gold leaf or silver leaf picking out subtle molding details.

Cabinetry

Square or arched-raised panel doorstyles in finishes similar to moldings would be used. Rich mahogany or cherry are also typical.

Countertops

Marble or granite with highly polished finishes, wood or ceramic tile are used, and solid surfacing, especially in stone-like patterns and colors.

Floors

Marble tile, especially black and white checkerboard patterns are used. Solid vinyl tile can reproduce a similar look. Hardwoods in parquet and intricate bordered patterns adorned with Oriental area rugs may be used for softness and color.

Furniture

Chippendale, "Chinoiserie," Sheraton, Hepplewhite or Queen Anne-type cabriole-legged tables and chairs ornamented with classical "shell" motifs would be typical, also upholstered wing chairs with ball and claw foot tables.

Fabrics

Rich silks, damasks, tapestries and brocades in deep, jewel tones are typical.

Wallcoverings

Patterns should be refined, like vertical stripes, elegant rich florals, swags, urns and ribbon motifs in very formal themes. Textured moiré or strie patterns. Chinese and Oriental motifs are popular, as well as classical patterns with festooned or draped swags. Elaborate fruity borders emphasize moldings in the kitchen.

Accessories

Blue willow plates, pagodas, pavilions and dragon images are found on china, fabrics and wallpaper. Chinese baskets, fine porcelain and delftware are used, as well as gilded mirrors, portraits and landscape paintings.

Classical fluted columns top an ornamental and crowned cornice fashioned out of gleaming, rich cherry wood, which houses the tub in this classically styled bathroom. ➔

Designed by Kalliroy Pappas, CKD; Photo by Maura McEvoy

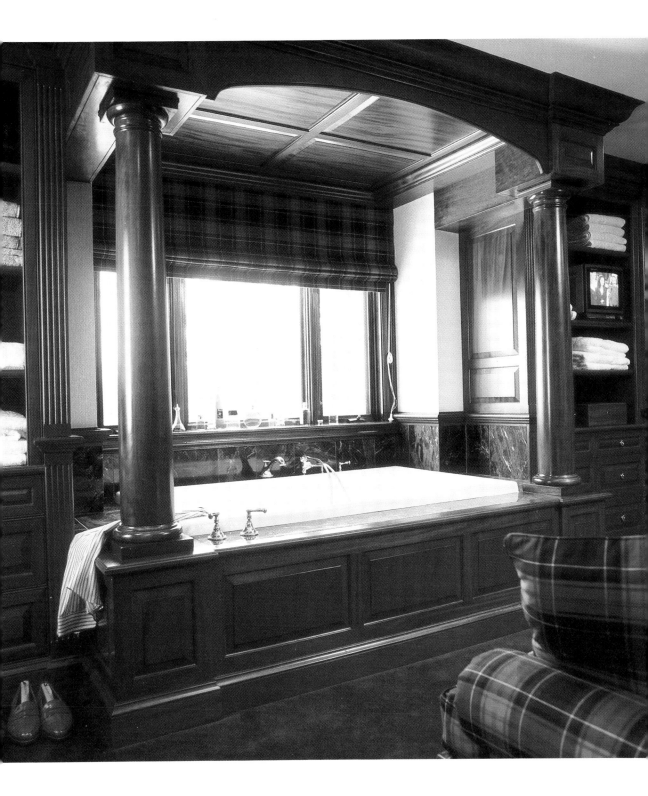

The Queen Anne "cabriole" furniture leg is adapted from the graceful lines of an animal's leg, hence the "claw" and "hoof" detailing at the foot.

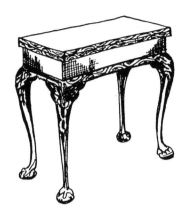

Typical fretwork "Chinoiserie" styling of the Georgian period.

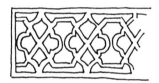   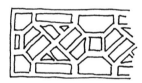

Decorative motifs derived from ancient Greek and Roman architectural ornamentation—egg and dart frieze pattern, dentil frieze pattern, Greek key frieze pattern and acanthus leaf.

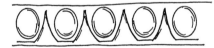   

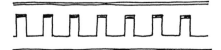   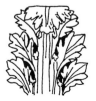

Courtesy of NKBA

Queen Anne and Early Georgian furniture styles.

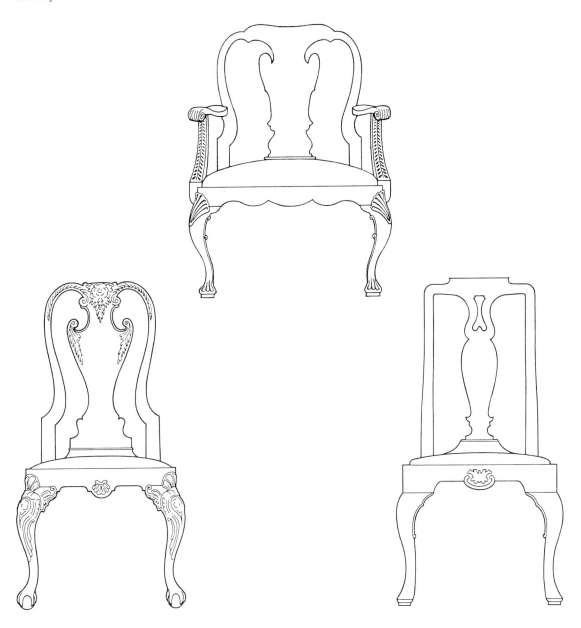

Queen Anne furniture styles typical of the classical Georgian styles, rather than the Victorian style of the same name.

Courtesy of NKBA

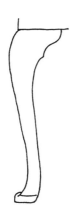

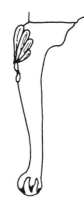

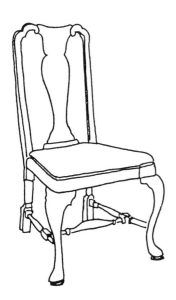

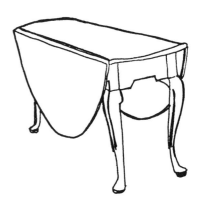

Georgian Chippendale furniture styles were Western interpretations of Oriental decorative styles and motifs.

Courtesy of NKBA

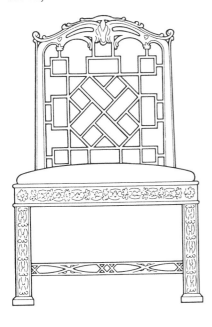

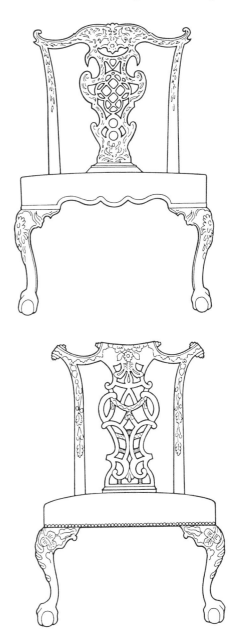

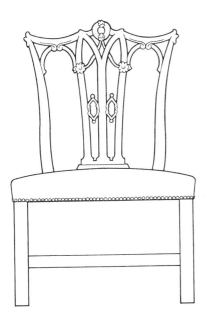

Adams and Regency styles of ornamentation for furniture.

Courtesy of NKBA

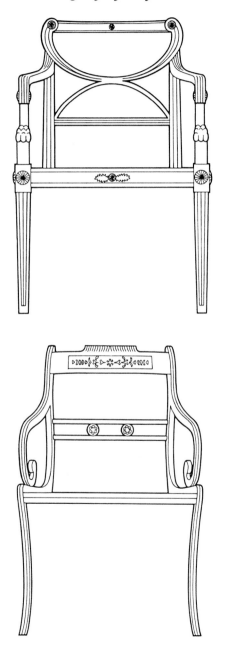
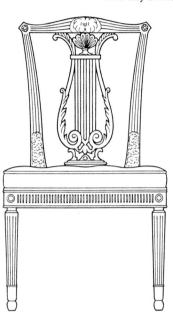
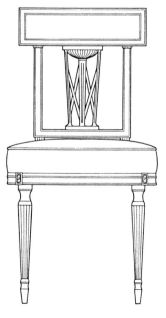

Courtesy of NKBA

Hepplewhite and Sheraton furniture styles.

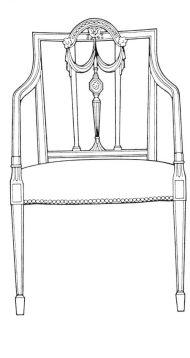

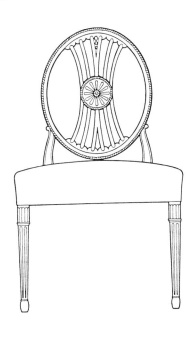

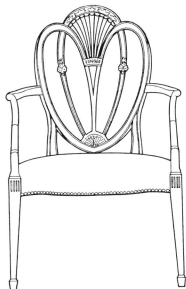

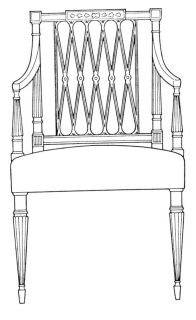

CLASSICAL
Neo-Classic/Greek Revival

Historic Context

Based on the architecture and interior design principles of Robert Adams, interiors of these homes actually go beyond classical Roman influences to incorporate Greek and Etruscan themes. It may be noted that the later Federal period styles were also greatly influenced by Napoleonic France.

Walls/Ceilings

Plain, plastered walls are set off with Ionic columns, pilasters, doorcases and deep cornices. Ceilings decorated with medallions, swags and ornate borders created out of plaster are important decorative elements. Subtle color schemes would be in pale greens, blues and pinks, or black and white, highlighted with gold leaf for a very formal tone. Dusty gray-greens or peach-creams are used for a lighter, less formal look. Faux-painted walls like rag rolling, strie (combing) or sponged color over color create a look of deep age.

Windows/Doors

Windows usually consist of larger panes of glass, not divided into mullions as in earlier styles. Symmetrical arrangement is still important.

Moldings

Moldings are bold and pronounced, but less massive and with more delicate detail than earlier Classic styles. Bas-relief urns have garland swags as a typical motif.

Cabinetry

Beaded inset paneled doors, with applied simple moldings in painted finishes of white, cream or dusty pastel tones are most common. Rich burgundy wood tones would also simulate the Duncan Phyfe and Sheraton furniture popular at the time. Woods would be mahogany, walnut and cherry.

*Greek Revival urn motif
typically found in ornamental
plaster detailing.*

Countertops

Laminates in stone-like patterns and colors, and solid surfacing
with classical, built-up edge details, possibly incorporating
contrasting edge striping, would be typical. Ceramic tiles with
delicate pattern designs or rich terra cotta colors are used as
accents.

Floors

Marble tiles, oiled floor cloths painted to resemble marble
patterns, and solid vinyl tiles would be used. Long strip wood
floors in maple, cherry, mahogany or white oak, with decorative
border striping and/or corner details, are other possibilities. Rich,
dark floors play off painted cabinets and woodwork in whites,
creams and peach tones.

Furniture

Period furniture employed the decorative use of shields, urns,
swags and eagles. Shield- or medallion-backed chairs are typical
of the Sheraton and Duncan Phyfe styles. Gold leaf medallion
details, Napoleonic motifs and gilt stars adorn bookcases, tall floor-
length "pier" mirrors fashioned in beautifully finished exotic
veneers. Greek key motifs, columns and pilasters are repeated in
furniture detailing, adapted from the architectural surroundings.

Fabrics

Damasks, silks, striped ticking, block-printed patterns on linen, velvets, woven tapestries, Fortuny and toiles are used. Chinese silks and printed patterns of stylized laurel wreaths, swags and the Napoleonic bee were popular.

Wallcoverings

Similar patterns to those found in fabrics suitable to the period, as well as faux textures and stries, are typical. Stripes in both high- and low-contrast color combinations are used.

Accessories

Wedgewood china, featuring Roman and Greek original pottery motifs, is one example of accessories. Bronze, silver, gilt and crystal accents add sparkle and interest. Blue and white pottery and figurines grace arched, recessed niches cased in shell-motif moldings.

Duncan Phyfe furniture.

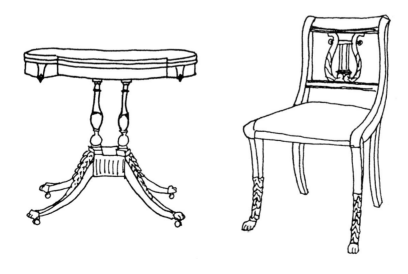

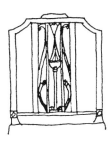
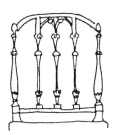

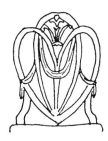
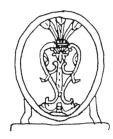

*Duncan Phyfe, Hepplewhite, "lyre" motif and
Sheraton "medallion backed" chair styles.*

The wall covering, pale wood tones and swagged window treatments are typical of the Neo-Classic Federal styles. The high contrast of black and white are formal Greek Revival influences.

Designed by Maria E. Weingard

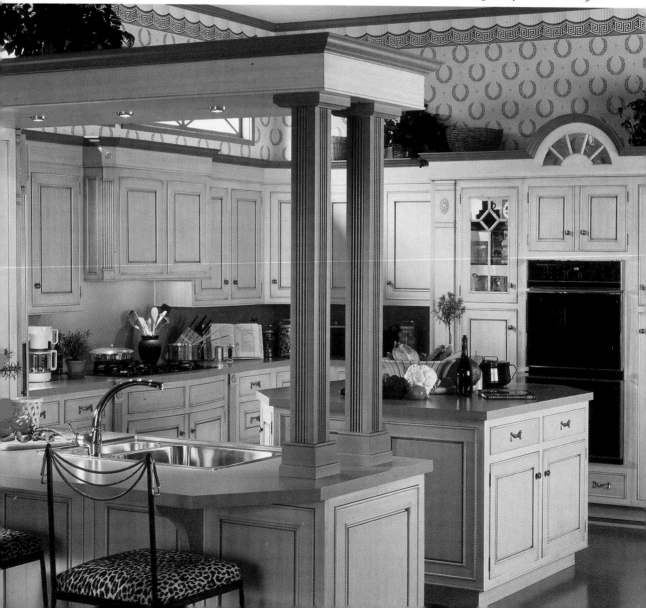

Designed by Maria E. Weingard

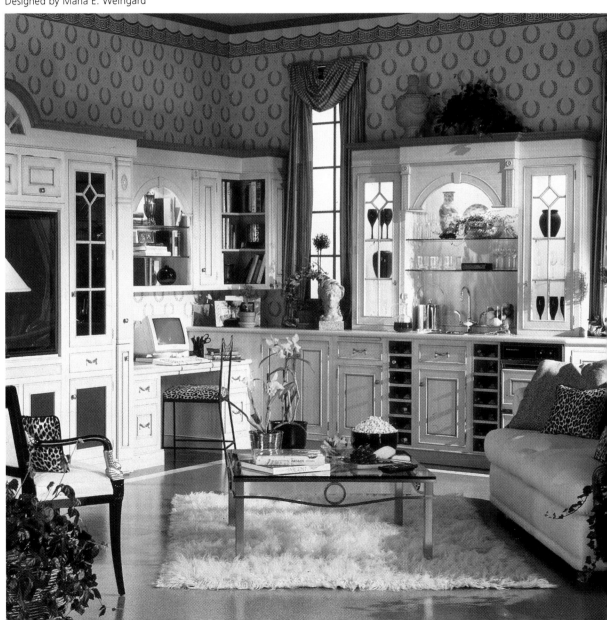

A Greek Revival swag and pale wood tones are combined with a more heavy-handed use of moldings, typical of classical Georgian theme.

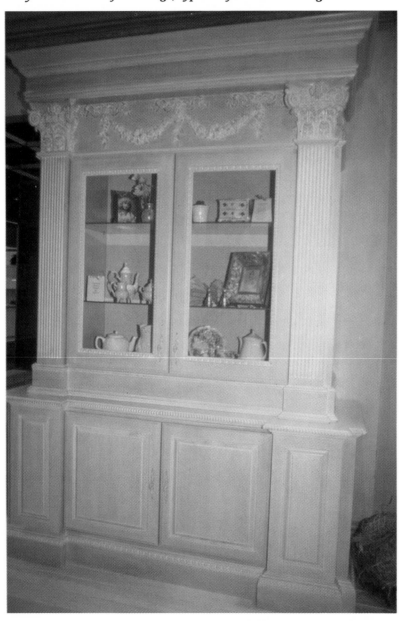

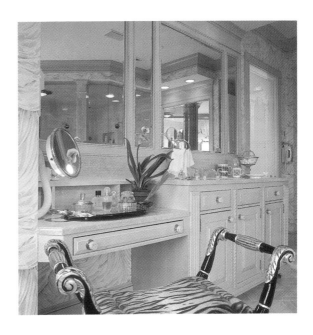

A Neo-Classic bathroom with marbled floors, heavy crowns, fluted columns and miles of swags. Pale monochromatic color scheme is punctuated by gilt and black enameled Roman Neo-Classic chair.

Designed by Thomas Kling, CKD; Photos by Maura McEvoy

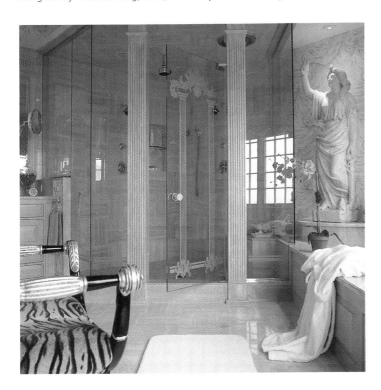

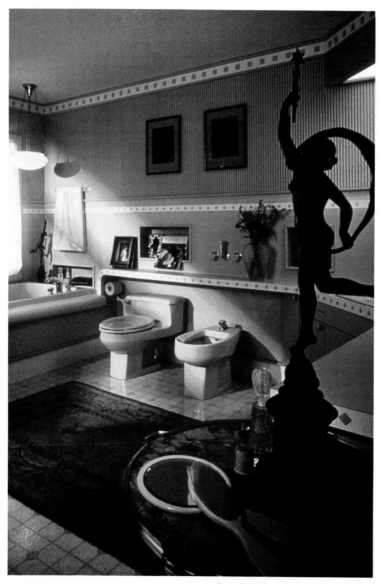

Courtesy of Wilsonart International

Neo-Classic bathroom in taupe, black and ivory composes a formal Greek Revival color scheme. Crown, chair rail and counter edge suggest a classical dentil mold. The pared-down simplicity of the ornamentation is Neo-Classic in spirit.

An example of high style Neo-Classic design. This bathroom combines marble floors, classically curved walls that are devoid of ornamentation and Roman-column pedestal lavs with a Roman-styled iron bench.

Courtesy of Kohler Co.

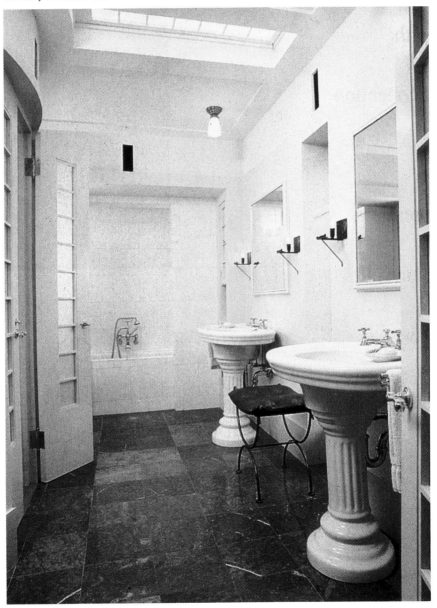

BARONIAL
Gothic Revival/Picturesque/Tudor Revival

Historic Context

The Early Gothic styles were inspired by the great baronial halls of the Middle Ages, where grand manor houses in rural settings demanded plenty of space and a wide, sprawling design. These themes contain reference to heraldry, royal courts and Knights of the Round Table.

Look for rollover of themes into the Victorian Styles. The Early Gothic interiors are characterized by overall use of pattern and texture. Medieval themes and influences, and romantic, sentimental notions of the Middle Ages and medieval chivalry, are also evident in these themes.

Walls/Ceilings

Rough plaster, sometimes paneled with "linenfold" oak paneling is used. Lancet arches and vaulting delineated by heavy beams and cross timbering define interior spaces. Brick and plaster walls can be limewashed white, or tinted earth colors in flat finishes, sometimes painted or stenciled with decorative motifs, such as

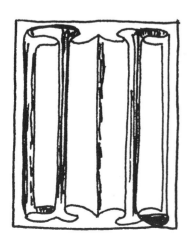

Linenfold paneling.

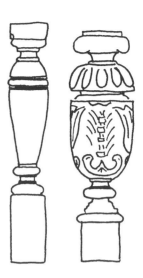

Heavily turned and carved table legs are typical of Baronial styling.

heraldic emblems or coats of arms. Ceilings could be painted fresco style, or with Gothic-patterned designs. Some wallpapers are especially designed for ceiling application, with stars, interlocking patterns, Gothic "tracery," trefoils and quatrefoils, all in small scale. Color schemes include matte red ocher, dusty pink, stone greens with gilt accents, rich reds and maroons, forest greens, yellows, ultramarine and verdigris.

Windows/Doors
Often diamond-paned, leaded glass, arched or both, windows were draped with heavy velvet or damask curtains hung from wrought-iron rods. Other wrought-iron work of truss braces, stair railings and brackets were typical.

Moldings
Gothic tracery in wood, iron or plaster would display intricate detail, with lacy, almost gingerbread trelliswork. Plaster moldings on walls could be highlighted with white or cream paint.

Cabinetry

Limed washes or rubbed aniline-tinted shellac, pickled pine, or dark antique oak are suitable. Also common was heavy, massive styling, either plank doors or square or recessed panels. If available, lancet arches could be incorporated on a few focal doors, as they would be quite evocative of the style. Leaded glass, in diamond patterns, would also be effective. Woods used were primarily dark, blackened oaks and pale, limed oaks.

Countertops

Limestone, slate or wood are used, with texture and age more important than color.

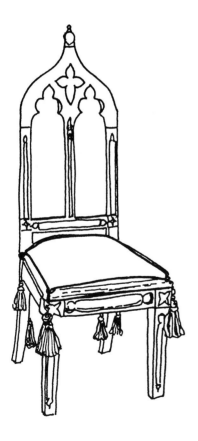

Gothic-styled chair with ecclesiastic details, tassels and quatrefoils.

A lancet-arched and diamond-paned window.

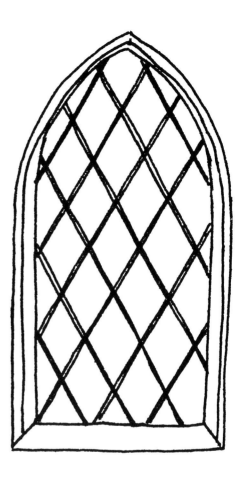

Floors

Dark stone, slate or wood are good choices. Ceramic tile in rustic pavers, giving a cobblestone effect, would work well. Wood floors may be stained in two-toned finishes to resemble combinations of oak and walnut, marble tiles, etc. Sisal carpeting, designed to resemble rush matting, and brick floors, especially in herringbone patterns combined with oak strips, are suitable for this theme. Plain, polished wood floors in medium to dark tones or in limed, antiqued finishes may also be used.

Furniture

Combinations of wood, wrought iron and marble are all common to the theme. Oak "Mission" style and Jacobean styles add a massive elegance. Furnishings are minimal and simple, which exaggerates a sense of volume and over-scale in rooms. Trestle tables, chests and benches with either woven rush or leather seats may be used.

Fabrics

Great woven wall hangings, typically tapestries, would soften the austere settings. Needlework or rich fabrics suspended by metal or wooden rods also work. Fabric patterns in fleur-de-lis, trefoils, quatrefoils, stars, quoins, crowns and royal motifs are typical, as are leather and faux animal skins.

Wallcoverings

Patterns and colors similar to fabrics can be used, as well as gilt, gold and silver leaf detailing, heraldic motifs, small, open patterns or gothic trelliswork. Rich detail with high definition, resembling tapestries, toiles and woven textures are typical. Mythical, magical and exotic themes are also appropriate.

Accessories

Small, dim lamps or candlelight, wrought-iron lamps with parchment shades, wooden or pewter dishes and bowls, shield designs and greenery such as topiaries are all possible choices.

VICTORIANS
High Victorian

Historic Context

Medieval motifs such as stylized floral patterns, filigree, lancet-arched windows and leaded glass windows are carried over from earlier styles to help create this intricately detailed theme. Victorian interiors are best described as eclectic and full of rich detail. High Victorian interiors are not for everyone, as is seen in this interesting quote from an interior design text of the 1930s, when Victorian interiors were a not too distant—and not too fond—memory:

> Who does not remember those old houses, the heavy, badly designed furniture, unsympathetic haircloth on sofas and chairs, requiring great knitted tidies to make it tolerable—the grotesquely colored and patterned carpet and aggravating wallpaper? The parlor—which was seldom used—with its graveyard pictures worked in hairwork, beads or embroidery, waxwork objects of art (?), safely set under a big glass bell, big boxes on the 'center table'—set exactly in the center of the room—holding boxes of ashes of the dear departed or faded flowers from the coffin. And the inartistic upholstery hiding its blushes under a profusion of crocheted antimacassars, reminding one of an eternal washing day. - Katherine Muselwhite, *The Principles and Practice of Interior Design*

Walls/Ceilings

Ceilings were richly decorated, with the addition of patterned tin ceilings and cornices. Walls most typically were papered. Strength of color is essential: gold, jade green, lily blue, green and cream combinations, peach, terra cotta, pink and green, copper, verdigris, black and white, lavender blues. In kitchens and bathrooms, beadboard paneling or tile wainscoting were typical.

Windows/Doors
Bay, bow and box bay windows are common, with abundant window treatments, often several layers at each window, hung from brass or wooden rods. Roller blinds under drapery treatments in cream or green are also typical.

Moldings
Fluted, flat-board trims at windows and doors with "bullseye" corner blocks are common. Tall, built-up base molding and patterned crowns and cornices in classical motifs are typical, except when combined without the reasoned order of the earlier classical periods.

Cabinetry
Painted or wooden cabinets with numerous glass inserts, built-in breakfronts, china cupboards and dressers with open shelves above are appropriate. Mixing finishes helps to achieve an unfitted, furniture look to focal pieces. Brass or glass hardware in clear or tinted finishes can also be used.

Countertops
Wood, marble, granite, stainless steel or ceramic tile, especially in 3 x 6 brick shapes, laid in running bond in white or ivory tones are suitable, in addition to Spode-like decal printed tiles in delicate, intricate patterns.

Floors
Marble, limestone or terrazzo are good choices. Similar patterned linoleums or vinyls are also satisfactory. Floral-patterned hook rugs and Oriental carpets add texture, color and pattern over hardwood floors.

Furniture
Mahogany, blackened oak, walnut, satinwood and rosewood pieces were mixed with wicker and papier mâché pieces to offset the heaviness of the wood and upholstered furnishings. Upholstery fabrics of wool, mohair, velvet, Oriental woven cloths and paisleys were common.

Fabrics

Patterned chintzes and lace can be added to the less formal rooms. In more masculine settings, tartans, heraldic emblems and leather would be suitable.

Wall Coverings

Wallpapers were first mass produced in the 1840s, making them available to the middle classes. Wallpapers, like carpets and fabrics of the period, were highly patterned and richly colored.

Glazed, flocked and gilded wallpapers were used in more formal settings. Embossed wallcoverings such as Lincrusta and Anaglypta were used on ceilings and below chair rails, usually painted in darker, leathery tones. Most rooms would have a chair rail with a different decoration below and above it, topped with a decorative frieze around the top of the wall.

Ceramic-tiled walls in kitchens and bathrooms were common, as a result of great concern for hygienic surfaces.

Accessories

Souvenirs of travel or exotic collections are used for display. Shells, boxes, silverware and porcelains are all suitable. Lots of books and architectural detail lend a scholastic, worldly air, while paintings in gilt frames, oils and watercolor landscapes, and elaborate botanical prints, are also desirable. Brass, marble, intricate metal scroll-work, Majolica pottery and Straffordshire china were popular during this period.

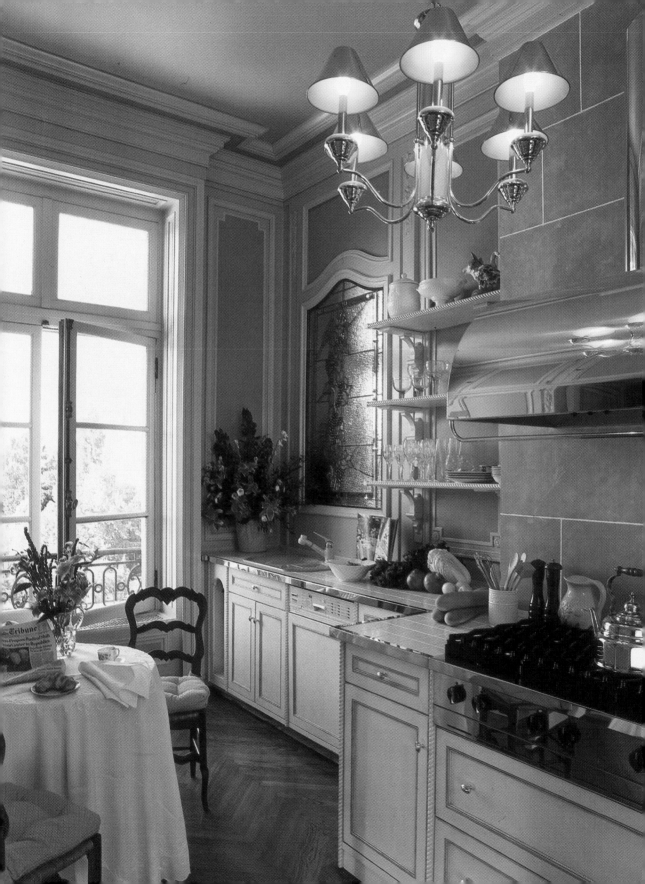

← *High Victorian style does not need to be dark to be successful. This beautiful Victorian kitchen combines pastels and light colors with bright brass accents, and rich herringbone parquet floors for a light-filled but elegant architectural space.*

Designed by Bernadine Leach and Peggy Deras, CKD

This Victorian kitchen combines many surface treatments—brick wall, papered walls and ceilings with dense, rich pattern, and color and tile patterned floor with Oriental rug. Cabinetry is configured to look like a piece of furniture with green marble top. Loaded with rich detail and texture.

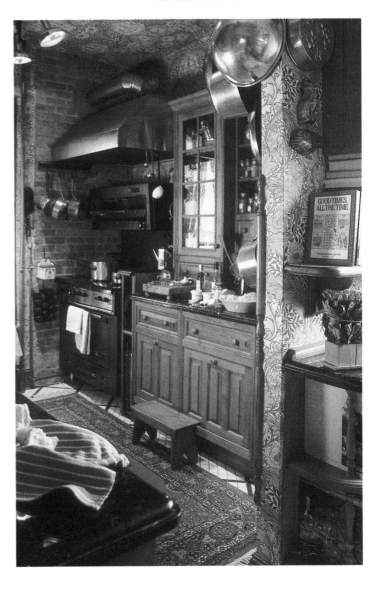

This Victorian-themed bathroom combines cabbage rose wallpaper, rich cherry cabinetry with marble, and bright brass accents for a formal, High Victorian look.

Designed by Deborah Schroll and Gordon Schroll

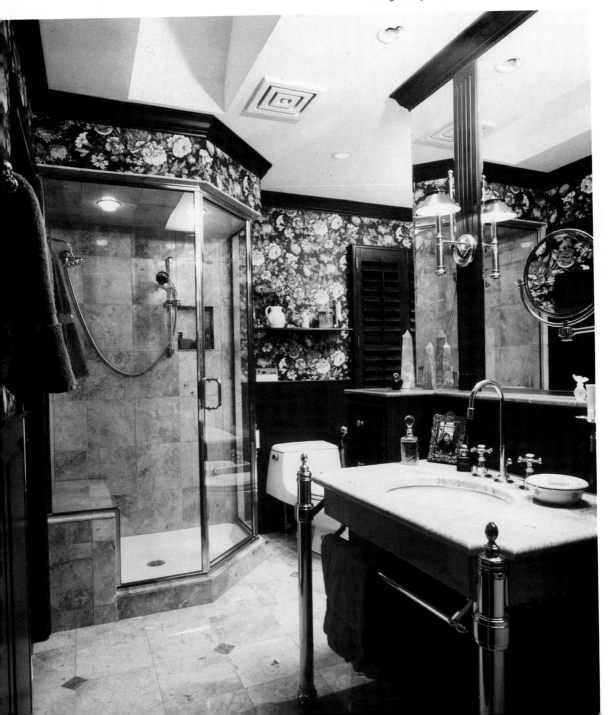

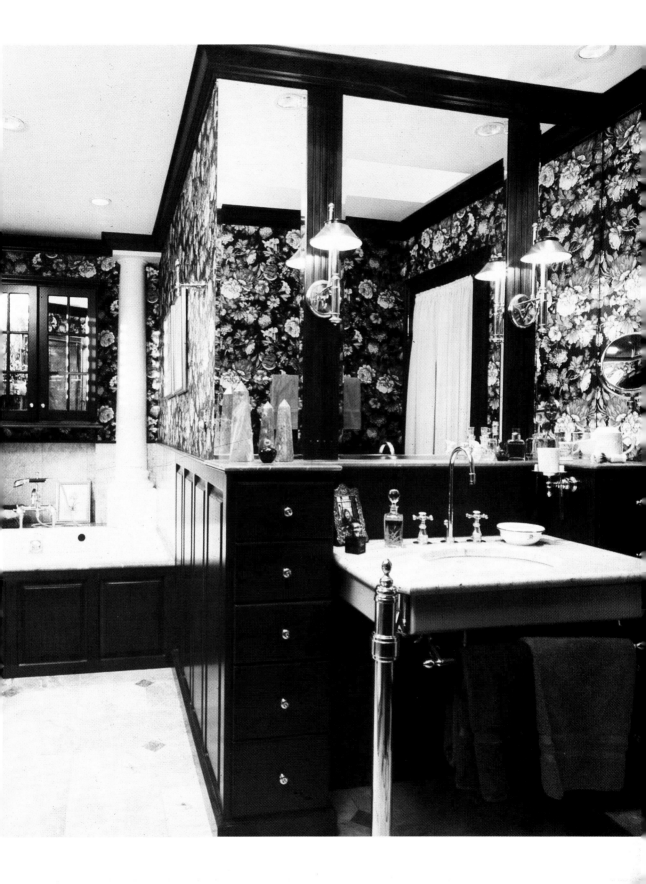

VICTORIANS
Queen Anne
(Informal Victorian)

Historic Context
Interiors in the Queen Anne style are much the same as the High Victorian style, but a little less formal and stuffy, with a more "cottage-y" and light-handed feel. Queen Anne interiors tend to have a relaxed informality about them, with a slightly worn and shabby edge that engenders a more comfortable, lived-in feel. Less heavy and cluttered than High Victorian interiors, this style leans toward the Arts and Crafts and English Country styles. These can be found mostly in country homes in rural or suburban settings, and in farm houses in Vernacular styles.

Walls/Ceilings
Walls were often painted light, sunny colors, or papered in flowery wallpaper. White and pastel shades are introduced, with occasional touches of darker greens, reds, blues or black. Generally, walls and ceilings are treated much the same as High Victorian, but are less formal.

Windows/Doors
Similar to High Victorian, but with some cottage-style elements of the Tudor styles mixed in. For example, diamond-paned leaded glass, or wood mullioned glass is typically used as a decorative element in this style. Also, decorative mullions used in the top half of double-hung sash windows in styles similar to patterns used in Arts and Crafts styles.

Moldings
Beadboard paneling, combined with painted or stained moldings, is common in kitchens and bathrooms.

Cabinetry

Cabinetry would have simple recessed panels, beaded inset doors, and sometimes sliding bypass doors. Modest decoration in the form of applied molding might be used. Unfitted designs combined with large, commercial appliances give a timeless quality.

Countertops

Ceramic tile, wood or wood-patterned laminates, linoleum, stainless steel would have been used, with pale marble or limestone in bathrooms. Solid-surface materials are present-day alternatives, especially in patterns resembling marble.

Floors

Wood plank floors were covered with rag rugs or striped cotton dhurries, or large Oriental carpets over sisal to resemble rush matting. Bathroom floors were often tiled, as were walls, with small hexagonal mosaic tiles, or black and white marble tiles. Solid vinyl tiles are a modern substitute.

Furniture

Queen Anne tables and Windsor chairs would look at home. Free-standing antique hutches, sideboards or dressers give rooms an antique presence and set the tone for other cabinetry.

Fabrics

Lace, muslin, chintz, quilts, linen and needlepoint are added to the usual Victorian mix.

Wallcoverings

Large-scale, flowery wallpaper in pale shades on white or cream backgrounds offer pattern and tone without closing a room in. Also, pinstripes, landscape borders and checks are common, often all mixed together, to create a carefree jumble of patterns and color. Also typical would be linen and jute fabric wall coverings.

Accessories

Iron and brass accents, wicker, verdigris metal finishes.

*Light-colored walls, simple glass-door cabinets, brass accents and
pastel colors sit comfortably and almost cozily on the black and white
harlequin-patterned floor. The black and white linoleum tiles mimic
marble tiles; this was an authentic design device of the era.*

Designed by Sherry A. Faure, CKD; Photo by David Livingston

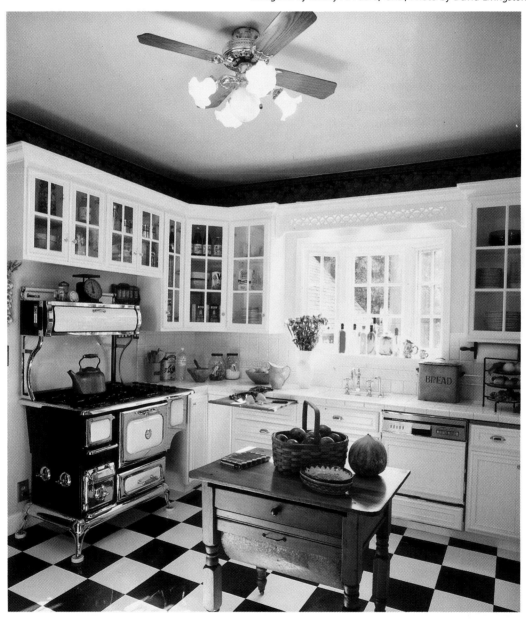

Two views of a Queen Anne Victorian style bathroom, with painted white cabinetry and woodwork, floral wallpapers in open, flowing patterns and an abundance of light.

Designed by William Earnshaw, CKD, CBD; Photo by Maura McEvoy

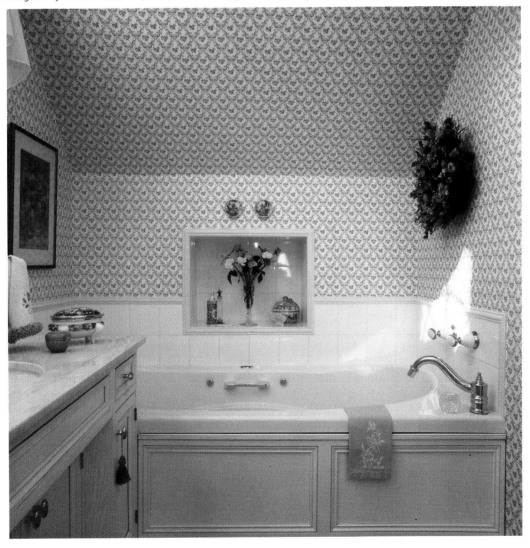

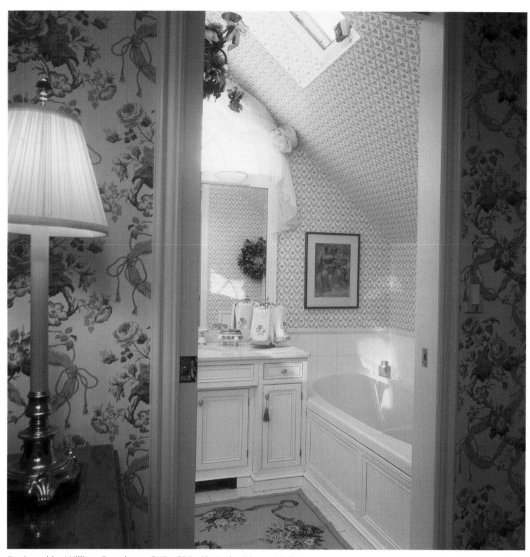

Designed by William Earnshaw, CKD, CBD; Photo by Maura McEvoy

This Victorian bathroom is almost Vernacular in its informality and rustic interpretation of Victorian design elements. It would be very much at home in a country farmhouse.

Photo courtesy of Kohler Co.

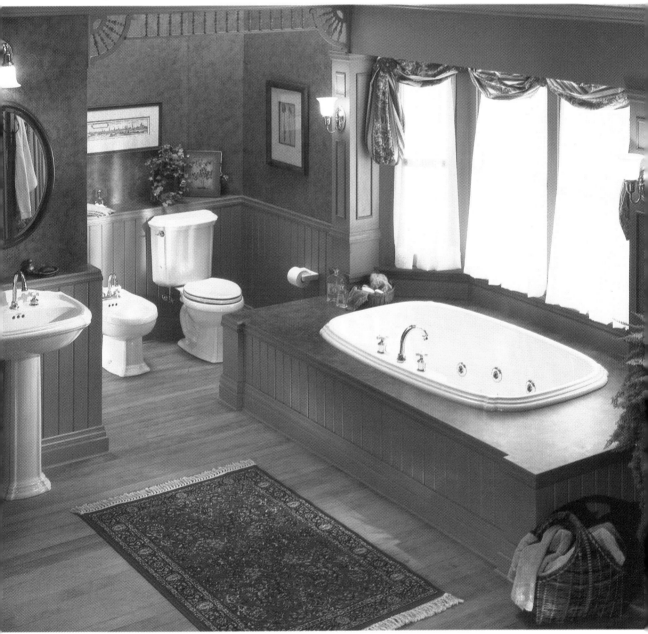

VICTORIANS
Edwardian
(Late Victorian/Early Art Nouveau)

Historic Context
Between 1901 and 1914, Victorian values and traditions mirrored the general acceptance of eclecticism in architecture and interior design. Luxury and comfort became higher priorities than the predominance of one style over another. Strong French influences appeared with the introduction of Parisian style and the beginnings of Art Nouveau. Arts and Crafts and Japanese elements are also discernible as influences of this style. Under close examination, it is easy to see a number of similarities to the English Country theme.

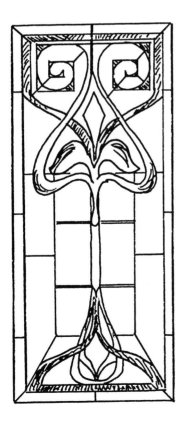

Edwardian decorative elements were almost Art Nouveau in their use of stylized natural motifs.

Walls/Ceilings

Mixed use of Georgian, Adams and Federal moldings and ornamentation without regard for symmetry and proportion was typical of each of these decorative styles. French classical decorative themes were also popular. Ceilings could be plaster, wallpaper or ornamental tin.

Windows/Doors

Decorative leaded-glass windows in stylized floral and natural motifs, typical of the Art Nouveau styles were used. Typically, glass is incorporated into doors or clerestory windows above to let in light.

Moldings

Door and window moldings are less formal than in earlier Victorian styles. Tudor- and Georgian-style paneling were also considered stylish. Delicately colored Minton tiles with border bands and skirting at baseboard trims were popular, especially in bathrooms.

Cabinetry

Tongue and groove paneled cabinet doors, punctuated with open ornamental shelving and glazed insert cabinet doors.

Countertops

Similar to earlier Victorian styles, both formal and informal.

Floors

The first inlaid linoleum patterns were used in this period, in colors and patterns designed to simulate more expensive floor coverings, carpets and wood. Parquet borders around fitted carpets of French and Persian design, and bordered carpets were popular. Pre-cut decorative parquet borders of elaborate patterns were available to inlay in hardwood floors. Mosaic tiled bathroom floors were still popular.

The curvilinear shapes combined with Craftsman-like simplicity suggest an Edwardian theme for this quietly elegant bathroom.

Courtesy of Kohler Co.

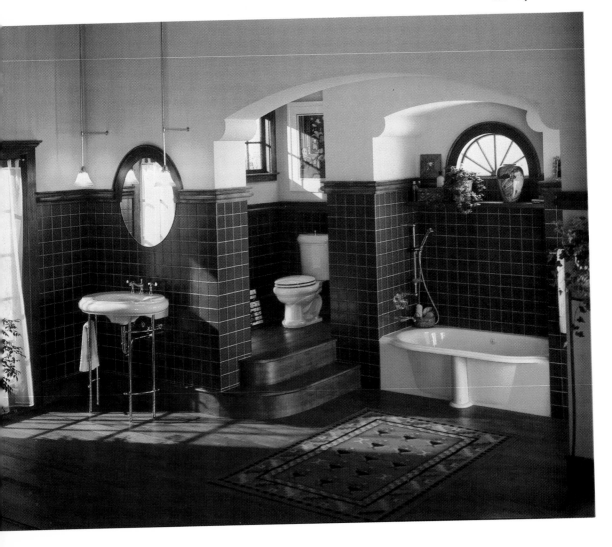

Furniture

Flowing Nouveau styles with simpler ornamentation in rich wood tones of cherry, mahogany and walnut. Fixtures began to be more streamlined and less convoluted in detail, as the ease of maintaining them became more important to the growing middle class. Victorian values and traditions continued along with a general acceptance of eclecticism in interior design. Luxury and comfort became higher priorities than the predominance of one style over another. Strong French influences are seen with the introduction of Parisian style and the beginnings of Art Nouveau. Arts and Crafts and Japanese elements are also discernible as influences of this style. There are many similarities to the English Country theme.

Fabrics

Fabrics were similar to Queen Anne styles. Curtains weren't typically used at windows in bathrooms, rather frosted, obscured or stained glass was used.

Wallcoverings

Wallpaper friezes and wallpapers with simulated fabric finishes like moiré, satin and stries were used extensively. Chintz-patterned papers with elaborate floral borders and embossed vellum paper on canvas backing that resembled fine wooden paneling were new introductions.

Accessories

Minton and Straffordshire china, bronze, silver, Japanese wooden boxes and ornaments, matte glazed pottery with Nouveau styling, flowing, delicate figurines, usually crafted in metal, were used. Books, gilt and hammered-metal picture frames, crystal, Oriental porcelain bowls and a profusion of flowers created busy tabletops.

This kitchen could be described as formal French Country, with the exception of the Georgian-styled moldings and fluted columns, and Nouveau curves in the glass doors and bar stools, which are more Edwardian in style.

Designed by Barton Lidsky

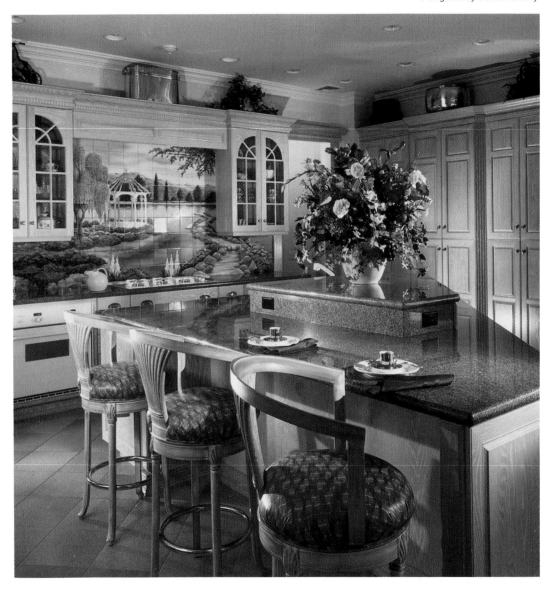

Designed by Barton Lidsky

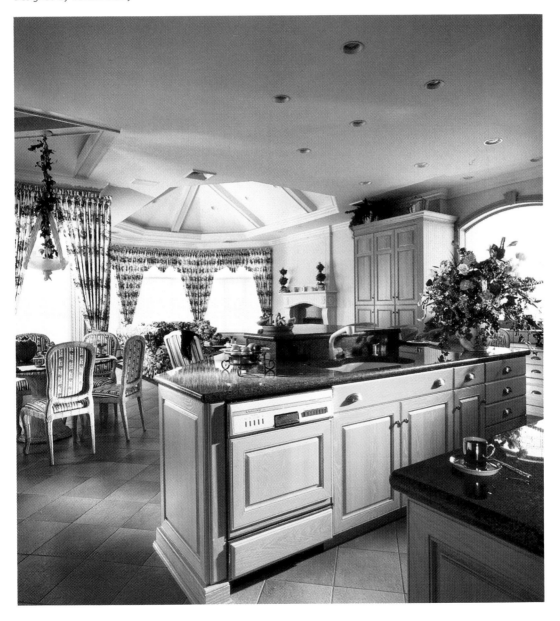

Luxury, Parisian influence and quiet sophistication make this a stand-out example of Edwardian style.

Designed by Gay Fly, ASID, CBD, CKD; Photo courtesy of Kohler Co.

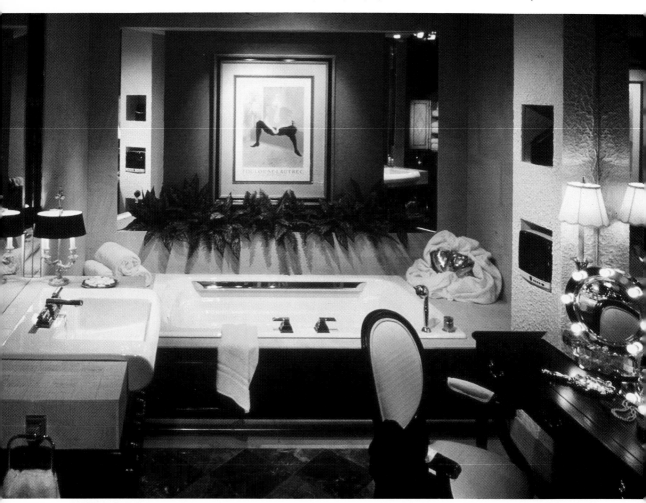

The beaded paneling, clerestory windows and blend of Victorian toward Craftsman elements could define this kitchen as Edwardian. The stylized natural motifs in the wallpaper and carpet help support the theme.

Designed by Cameron Snyder, CKD; Courtesy of Country Home Magazine

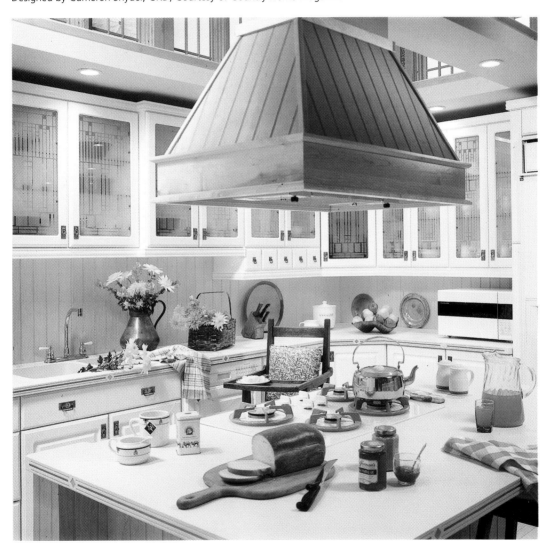

*The stylized wrought iron and marble of this console
vanity set the stage for an Edwardian-themed bathroom.*

Courtesy of Kohler Co.

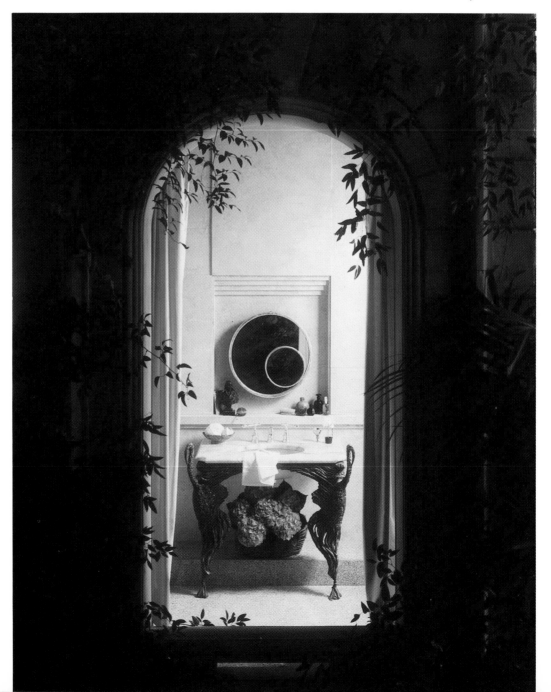

BAROQUE
Picturesque/Gothic/Tudor

Historic Context

Most closely associated with the Picturesque architectural styles, Gothic Revivals and Romanesque, this theme harks back to grand-scale structures which often resembled stone castles. The Baroque theme is best summed up by the word "decorum," the Latin word for appropriateness. Accordingly, in this style, classical orders of ornament are strictly applied and the proper use of ornament becomes of paramount concern.

Walls/Ceilings

Walls are paneled, sometimes faux painted to resemble marble or tortoiseshell. Ceilings were not usually plastered, but decorated with chamfering beams. Later, plaster ornament was used to emulate ancient architecture with grand cornices and friezes.

Windows/Doors

Diamond-paned casements and two-story bays resembling turrets provide stunning focal points and architectural form.

Moldings

Classical orders of ornament are strictly applied and the proper use and proportion of ornament is emphasized. Stairs and railings were massive in great halls with Jacobean-turned leg balusters. Ornate cast-iron railings, displaying metal filigree, were also used. Newel posts were heavily carved, sometimes into human forms, and this heavy carving was often carried out onto fireplace surrounds as well.

Cabinetry

Much the same as in Tudor and Gothic styles, but even more ornamented, cabinetry would be adorned with carved moldings that would integrate into door and window casings. Cabinetry designed to resemble furniture, such as china cabinets, buffets and armoires, can be used effectively as focal points in kitchens and bathrooms in this theme. Of course, fireplaces in kitchens or bathrooms would be highly desirable.

This heavily ornamented kitchen could be found in a castle. The lime-washed finish adds an aged, antique quality to the room.

Photo courtesy of Kathleen Donohue

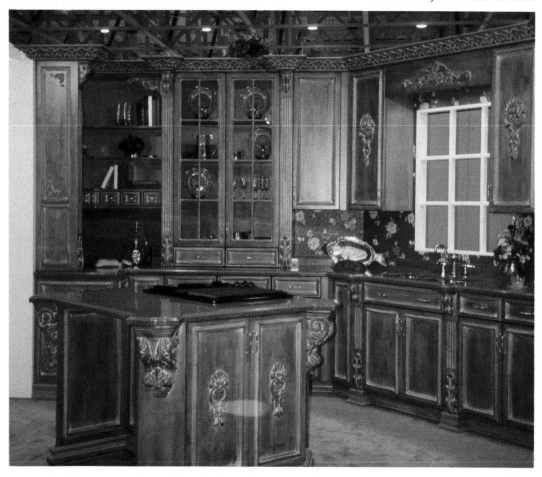

The "Gilded Age" is evoked with the heroic fireplace mantel, marble, rich wood tones, Ionic-fluted columns and crystal chandelier in the sumptuous interior.

Designed by Thomas Trzcinski, CKD, CBD and John Petrus; Photo by Julie Mikos

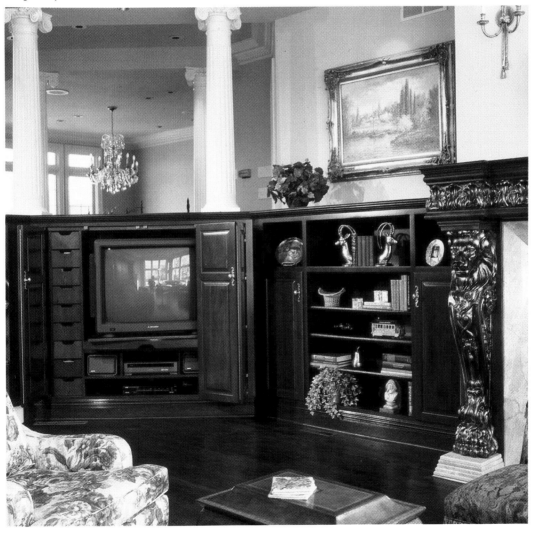

Countertops

Laminates that resemble stone, hammered copper or slate would provide a suitably rustic and textured effect. Ceramic tiles often displayed medieval motifs, such as heraldic designs, and were usually glazed in matte tones with rustic, handmade irregularities. Solid surfacing materials, dark or veined to resemble marble and combined with heavy, built-up edges, would also look and perform well.

Floors

Stone flags, brick or tile are typical, but marble and lime-washed wooden boards, patterned woods like parquetry and marquetry are also suitable. More common woods were often stained to look like walnut, mahogany and exotic woods. Woven carpets were typically Mediterranean in style, and placed beneath prized furniture. Also, they could be draped over tables, being considered too precious to walk on.

Furniture

Heavily carved antiques, loaded with ornamentation, were typical in the castle-like great halls, but Jacobean and rectilinear Mission styles also complement the look.

Fabrics

Tapestries, leather, brocades, fine linens and silks combine to give rich texture and jewel-tone color combinations.

Wallcoverings

Not as common as in other styles, except on ceilings and in alcoves, wallcoverings would be in parchment tones with gilt highlights in small-scale heraldic patterns or formal brocade and stripes.

Accessories

Added elements that suggest the feel of a grand hunting lodge, with artwork, trophies, alcoves and niches for built-in cabinetry and heavily carved brackets, would be used. In the bathroom, open, visible displays of towels, linens and bath oils suggest the splendor of a large manor house bath. Clawfoot tubs, or tubs built into ornate wooden pedestals filled with brass or gold faucets are in keeping with the theme. Towel warming bars, antique washstand and shaving mirrors add sparkle and give depth to the look.

The grand scale of classical ornament in this kitchen combined with the "aged" faux finish on the cabinetry give this kitchen a Baroque theme style.

Courtesy of Amana Appliances

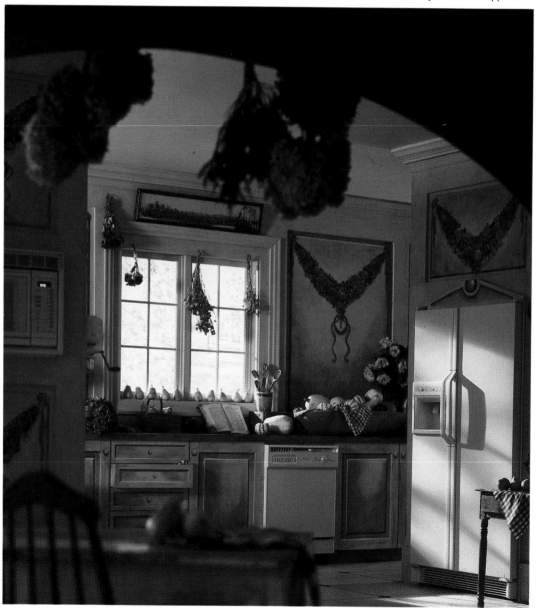

AESTHETIC
Art Nouveau

Historic Context
A post-Victorian style, the Art Nouveau theme was actually a precursor to the Arts and Crafts movement. Part of this movement can be attributed to Scottish architect Charles Rennie Macintosh, who designed furnishings and interiors to enhance and complete his designs. However, the Art Nouveau style also incorporates heavy influences from France, Belgium and Germany, utilizing furniture and fashion designs of stylized natural forms. These include flowers and a variety of curvilinear shapes much simplified from earlier Victorian excesses, often overlapping Edwardian styles.

Art Nouveau encompasses two different forms—one based on elongated, rectilinear forms with tight, precise floral ornament, and the other composed of wild, flowing, curvilinear elements characterized by a restless "whiplash" line. In many Craftsman homes, Art Nouveau elements were blended in to produce a more modern effect. Tiffany glass is the best example of true Art Nouveau form. Slightly curving vertical lines, suggesting plant forms, grids and curves, create rooms of austere elegance, with a clean, sparse beauty suggesting Japanese design elements.

Walls/Ceilings
White walls were not common, but instead often were lightly color-washed to relieve a perceived coldness in tones of cream or gray-blues. Muted greens, mauve, muddy browns, verdigris, bronze, silver and gilt, ocher creams, blue-grays and pale purples were fashionable. There should be an emphasis on integrated design, with wall treatments often carried up onto the ceilings, carrying the motif from vertical to horizontal.

Windows/Doors
Windows were treated with very simple, straight drapes crafted from elegant and rich textiles. Venetian blinds and roller shades were common "under treatments."

Moldings

Dark polished wood and metalwork of all kinds were used. Woodwork was either dark toned or black, or painted ivory white, revealing molding profiles and fretwork.

Cabinetry

Cabinet doors would be simple frame and recessed panel with art glass inserts for accent, or tooled copper. Painted finishes or natural wood tones of cherry, beech, mahogany, teak or walnut were used. Simple lines would be set off by carved curvilinear moldings or fretwork cutouts. Sometimes ebonized oak would be used for accent.

Spare, curvilinear design dominated Art Nouveau furniture design.

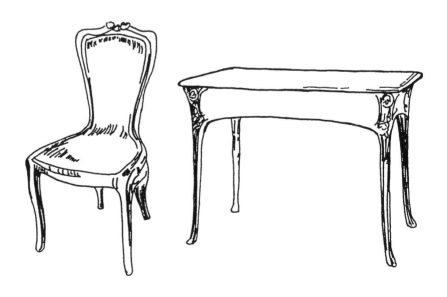

Countertops

Ceramic tiles would be muted jewel tones or slightly iridescent luster glazes. Wood, deep marble tones or rustic tumbled marble or limestone were also used.

Floors

Polished wood, often parquet, and ceramic tile were typical.

Furniture

Macintosh designed furnishings and interiors enhanced and completed his designs. Interiors were also heavily influenced by France, Belgium and Germany, incorporating furniture and fashion design of stylized natural forms. Art Nouveau encompasses two different forms—one based on elongated rectilinear forms with tight, precise floral ornament, and the other composed of wild, flowing curvilinear elements characterized by a restless "whiplash" line. Elements of Art Nouveau and Arts and Crafts were often blended together to create a pleasantly modern effect instead of completely radical interiors composed of these curving and undulating lines, which was a more flamboyant decorative effect and less common in homes. Rooms of austere elegance with clean, sparse beauty sprinkled with Japanese design elements sum up the look.

Fabrics

Printed and woven fabrics in stylized natural forms, silks, linens and ethereal gauzes were combined for texture and muted blends of color.

Wallcoverings

Wood paneling and tile wainscoting were used, creating a repeated pattern or one long motif, suggesting an undulating rhythm, as well as tile friezes and wallpapers. Favorite themes would be stylized flowers, sea plants, birds, peacock feathers—all

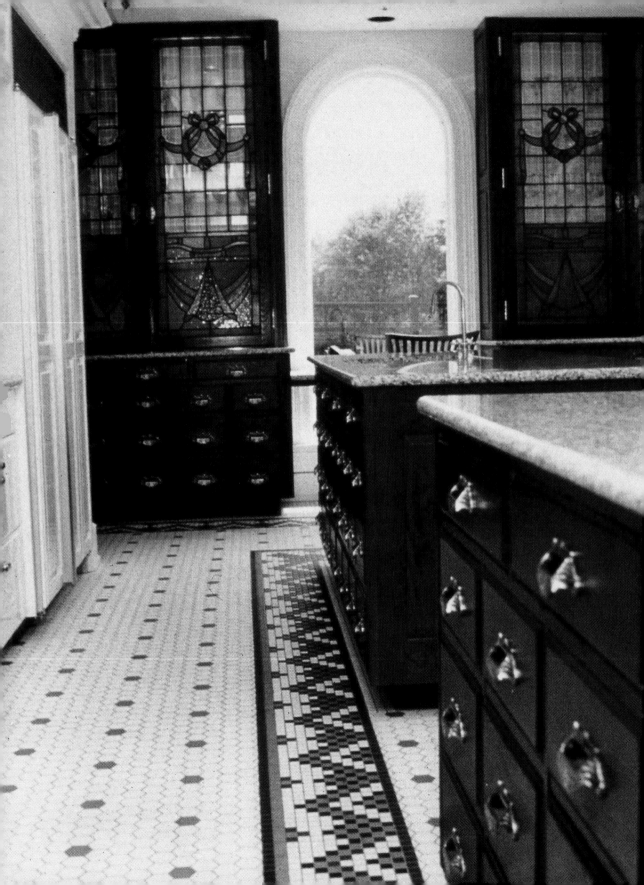

← *The straightfor-*
ward and simply
styled cabinets show
off the Art Nouveau
stained glass
inserts, letting them
make the design
statement for this
lovely kitchen.

Designed by T. Daniel Johnson

The curved forms and stylized natural motif of
the leaded glass panel manipulate this almost
Victorian bathroom into Art Nouveau style.

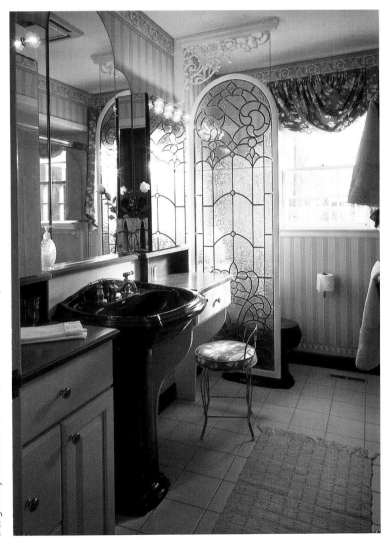

Designed by Richard M. Rawson, CKD, CBD; Photo by Sean Cranor

Art glass and brilliantly lustered ceramics carried out the theme of stylized natural forms to the smallest detail.

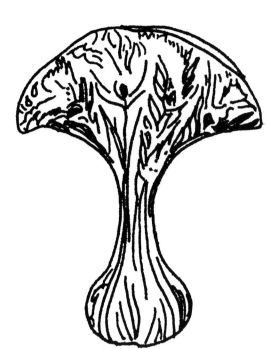

printed in rich colors. Ceiling papers in swirling, Art Nouveau patterns were designed to coordinate with wall patterns. In the bathroom, aquatic plant motifs, such as water lilies and lotuses were typical and even carried to the plumbing fixtures and tiles which were decorated in the same manner.

Accessories

Ceramics were finished in brilliant lusters, such as iridescent glassware. Artistic metalwork was crafted in brass, copper, silver or wrought iron. Tiffany glass is the best example of the Art Nouveau form, with slightly curving vertical lines suggesting, but not imitating, plant forms.

AESTHETIC
Biedermeier

Historic Context

Biedermeier finds its roots in a bourgeois style of furniture, art glass and ceramics that originated in Austria and Germany after the Napoleonic Wars. Probably a reaction to the Empire and Regency styles of France, this style is simplified but sophisticated, emphasizing geometric forms and classical motifs. Considered a sophisticated interpretation of Neo-Classic style, Biedermeier focuses on simple ornamentation and form and line, placing more emphasis on function and comfort than on flamboyance. Although it first occurred much earlier in the French Regency period, this style is generally grouped with the modern themes due to its clean, sharp forms, which blend well in a more contemporary or Neo-Classic setting. The strong contrasts of dark and pale woods are its hallmark.

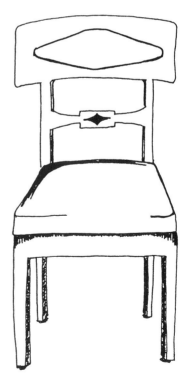

The classic lines of Biedermeier furniture were pared down and reduced to almost geometric elements. Pale wood was ornamented with dark ebony accents to emphasize the clear lines of the style.

Walls/Ceilings

Subtle beige, cream, vibrant yellow, blue, soft gray, aquamarine, sandstone and parchment with black and gilt accents were typical. High ceilings gave rooms a sense of generous proportion.

Windows/Doors

Simple, swagged window treatments, Roman shades, or wide venetian blinds are used.

Moldings

Classical moldings in clean, spare and simplified forms, incorporating high contrasts of ebony and pale wood tones. Many forms are similar to Greek Revival, but less ornamented and of simpler, flowing lines. Window and door moldings became wider and flatter. Definitely a very sophisticated look.

Cabinetry

Simple, clean lined "clair bois" (clear wood) styles consisting of pale tones of maple, beech, ash, pear and cherry with beaded inset panel, possibly set off by a black bead trim.

Countertops

Marble, granite, limestone or solid surfacing are used to play off the high contrasts of light and dark tones.

Floors

Bare woods and parquets are often outlined or bordered in ebony and set against walls painted in pale colors.

Furniture

Originally a bourgeois style of furniture and accessories that originated in Austria and Germany after the Napoleonic Wars. Biedermeier style was a reaction to Empire and Regency styles of France. The style is simplified and sophisticated, emphasizing geometric forms and classical motifs. A Neo-Classic style, focusing on form and line and simple ornamentation, placing more importance on function and comfort than grandeur and

Geometric forms and classical motifs are combined in this Biedermeier styled bathroom, along with the ubiquitous black accents added for high contrast.

Courtesy of Kohler Co.

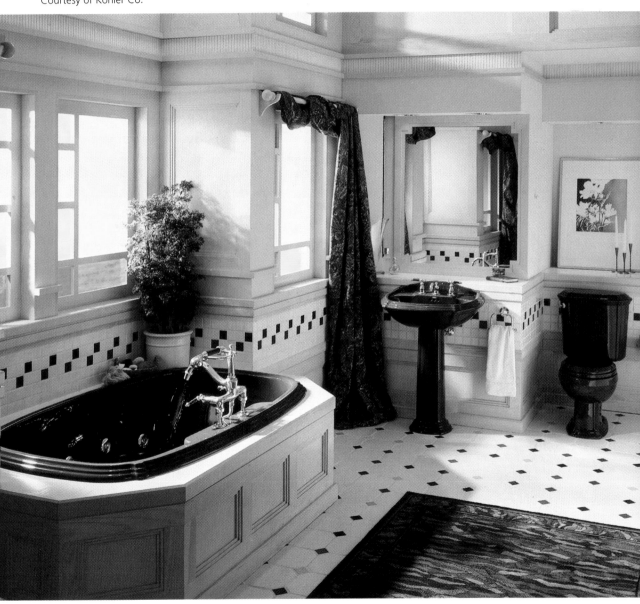

flamboyance. The strong contrasts of dark and pale woods are its hallmark. Curved lines of legs and chair backs combine with straight, rectilinear simple forms.

Fabrics

Leather, mohair, woven textures, small geometric prints and solid textures often trimmed with deep fringe and draped in classical swags.

The clean, spare lines, high contrast and geometric, but classical patterning of the marble walls in this bathroom would be suitable for a Biedermeier-themed room.

Designed by Tom Trzcinski, CKD, CBD

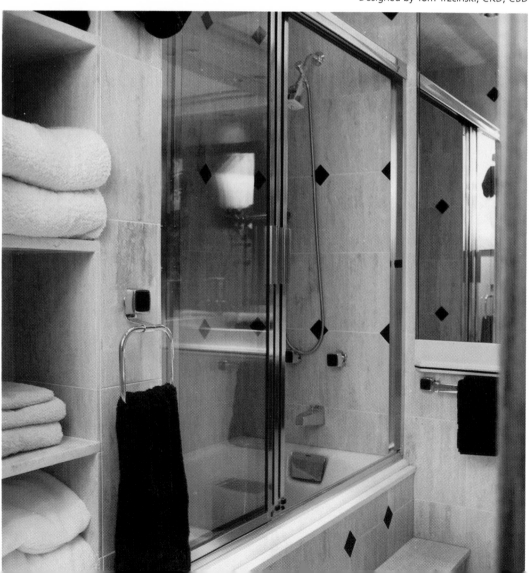

Wallcoverings

Small scale, finely detailed patterns, often finished at the top, bottom and sometimes in the corners with a gilt wood or metal fillet. Wallpaper borders in classic motifs were also common.

Accessories

Accessory choices include classical urns, gilt medallions and silhouettes.

Designed by Tom Trzcinski, CKD, CBD

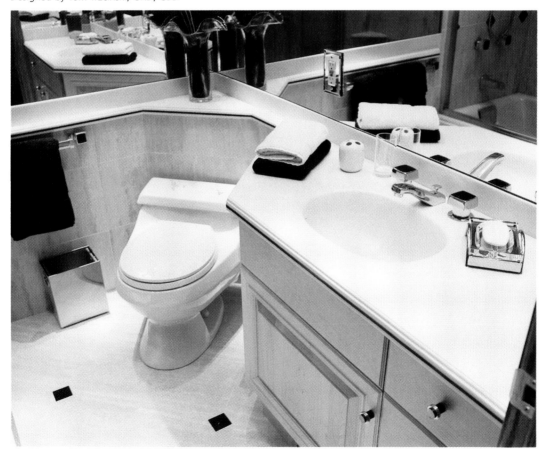

RUSTIC

Craftsman
(Arts and Crafts)

Historic Context

With strong roots in Tudor styles, the earliest Arts and Crafts designers in England were known as Medieval Revivalists. They idealized the rural, pastoral lifestyles of the villages of old England, as well as the fine craftsmanship and the medieval system of craft guilds, where handcrafted goods were highly prized. This was in sharp contrast to the low-quality products churned out by the industrial urban centers.

The traditional English Country cottage is considered to be the inspiration of the Arts and Crafts movement, following the general rules of the country builder, which stressed common sense and the use of locally available materials and building techniques.

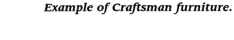

Example of Craftsman furniture.

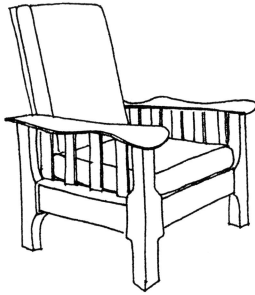

In addition to the strong English influence of the style, there are links to many other ethnic styles within the Craftsman genre. Simplicity and craftsmanship of the Shaker and pre-industrial Japanese arts were prized and collected. The Swedish Country style, made popular by artist Carl Larsson, had many parallels with Arts and Crafts tenets. Oriental themes, the stylized natural forms found in Chinese painting and the geometric woven textiles of India were collected and copied.

Another example of Craftsman furniture.

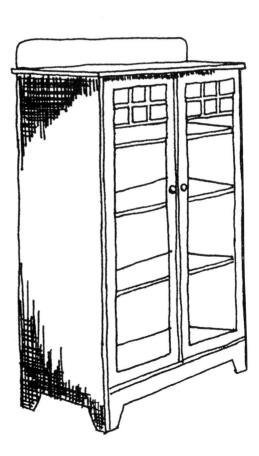

Reproduced from an issue of The Craftsman Magazine, this illustration depicts an ideal Craftsman kitchen as described by Gustav Stickley.

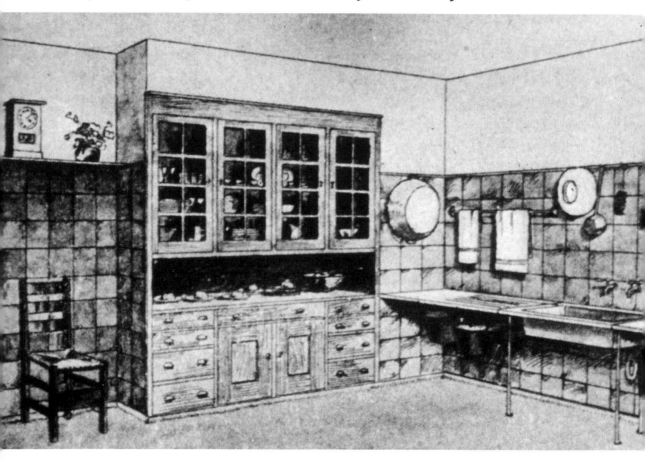

Crafts of the American Indian were also incorporated into many interior schemes. Even the folk and peasant crafts and lifestyles of Germany and Eastern Europe found their way into the Craftsman movement. The unifying theme of the Craftsman style is based on the concept of purity in both purpose and production techniques.

Walls/Ceilings

Walls were typically paneled up to about 5-feet high, and topped with a shallow shelf or plate rail. The plastered walls above the paneling were either painted or papered. Simplified timbering, usually with vertical and horizontal flat boards, was reminiscent of medieval construction and decor. In kitchens and bathrooms, walls were often tiled up to 5 feet, then also topped with a shelf or plate rail. Ceilings were rarely vaulted, but rather flat and low with box beams and coffering. Greens, muddy earth colors, natural wood tones, stone grays and browns, grayish blues and ocher yellow-golds were all fashionable.

Windows/Doors

Much the same as Queen Anne and Tudor Revival styles, windows are often grouped in horizontal bands, with double-hung sash windows having simple decorative mullions in the upper half only. Glazed French doors would typically not have divided lights. Other interior doors would be simple frame and recessed panels. Entrance doors would be wide, heavy timbered, often incorporating decorative glazing.

Moldings

Simple flat moldings at windows and doors, with top cross piece delineated by a ¼" - ⅜" parting bead and topped with a small scale crown. Baseboards would be simple 1" x 6" or 1" x 8" with base shoe trim, and sometimes topped with a small cove or ogee. Any ornamentation that is unnecessary would be eliminated. Clean lines, fine grains of wood and skillful joinery would take precedence.

The commercial-styled range fits beautifully into this no-nonsense Craftsman kitchen. Natural cherry cabinets, simply styled with understated moldings and the use of natural materials are unmistakable elements of the Craftsman style.

Designed by Alan Asarnow, CKD CBD; Photo by Maura McEvoy

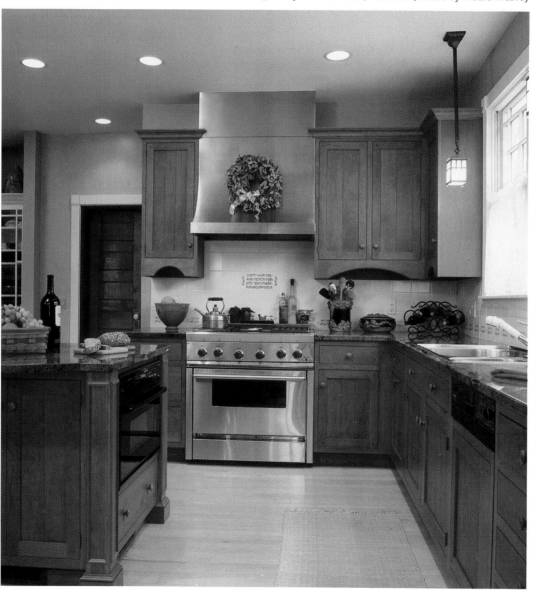

The nook incorporates use of typical Craftsman 5-foot height paneling, topped with a small ledge or plate rail.

Designed by Alan Asarnow, CKD, CBD; Photo by Maura McEvoy

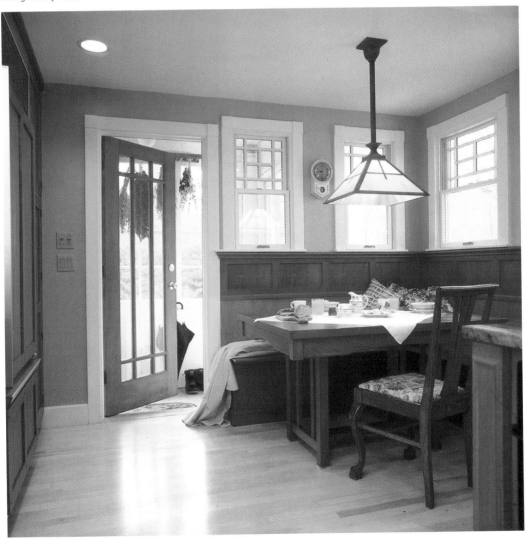

Cabinetry

Cabinet styling would be simple, as in the example of Craftsman furniture, in which the grain of the wood, joinery and hardware are the only decoration. Original Craftsman cabinetry was most likely painted, with simple square-edged frames and recess panels, but naturally finished fir, cherry, mahogany and quarter-sawn white oak would also be appropriate. Scrutiny of other woodwork in a vintage bungalow house that may have escaped the painter's brush can determine companionable wood species to use. Painted cabinets are not limited to white; creamy yellows, pale greens and French grays were all popular Craftsman colors and should be considered.

Countertops

Countertops can be made of wood, natural stone, granite, slate, soapstone and ceramic tile. Even plastic laminate or solid-surface materials that come in stone or wood patterns would look good and perform well.

Floors

Floors would generally consist of oak or fir, linoleum, ceramic tile, slate or flagstone, covered with American Indian woven rugs, flat woven dhurrie rugs or handcrafted loomed carpets. In the kitchen, flooring could be as simple as pulling up the old linoleum to reveal original fir or pine subfloors that could be sanded and refinished. Otherwise, true linoleums or vinyls in vintage patterns and matte finishes would be authentic. In the bathroom, ceramic tile floors and wainscoted walls are most typical, but vinyl and linoleum make good flooring choices.

Furniture

One of the most identifiable elements of the style is the furniture, which is known for its straightforward, unadorned lines, heavy horizontal and vertical masses and straight edges, relieved only by subtle curves. The grain of the wood, the artful joinery and the handcrafted hardware were its only adornment. A uniquely

American look, typical Craftsman furniture featured square spindles or slats, tapered legs, quadralinear, dovetailed construction, keyed and blind tenon and complicated butterfly joints. Larger cabinet and furniture such as armoires, sideboards, dressers and settees feature recessed inset panels and chunky corbels. Hardware was made of handcrafted metals with back plates, and hinges were often strap type. Wicker and peeled willow tables and chairs were often introduced to relieve the otherwise heavy furnishings.

Fabrics

Popular fabric looks included leather, wool, linen, woven tapestries, solid colors, geometrical and indigenous patterns and stylized florals.

Wallcoverings

Wallpaper friezes, especially landscapes and decoratively printed quotations and slogans, in the manner of medieval illuminated texts, were popular. Wallpapers were also stylized natural motifs in muted earth tones and were at once, Medieval, Oriental and Art Nouveau in their themes.

Accessories

Frequently used accessories included finely crafted items of wood, copper, clay, textiles, brass and iron. Medieval, Oriental and American Indian themes were all collected. American craft guilds, such as Roycrofters, Arequipa Pottery and Roseville Ceramics, all produced fine quality decorative objects that are highly collectible even today. Shaker baskets and boxes also work well in this theme style. Old world Japanese ceramic and metal crafts, woven textiles and baskets can be used to complete the look. The overall unifying theme of the Craftsman style is using elements with purity in both purpose and production techniques.

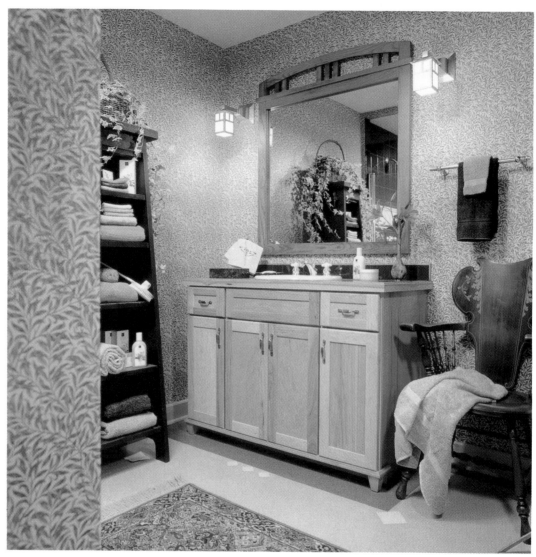

Designed by Cameron Snyder, CKD; Courtesy of Country Home Magazine

A William Morris print wallpaper featuring a stylized natural motif sets the tone in this Craftsman-themed bathroom.

RUSTIC
Lodge

Historic Context

This theme style has roots in the Arts and Crafts philosophy that advocates a return to nature and a desire for a simpler, more rural lifestyle. First associated with camps and lodges in the Adirondacks, this style was also popular in the western states and in the Southwest. Adopted by the U.S. Forestry Service during the Great Depression, this style can be seen in a number of public and service buildings in national parks. Hallmarks of this style include rustic pole furnishings, local river rocks and heavy timber framing.

Walls/Ceilings

Common were exposed log or plank walls, heavy plaster, often with wood cross members exposed. In the kitchen and bathroom, rustic ceramic tiles, bead-board paneling, natural and painted woods all work. Materials were used that made sense for the geographic region. Large, massive fireplaces and hearths, often with incorporated seating, were usually crafted from river rock or stone indigenous to the area.

Windows/Doors

Windows would be large and plentiful, consisting of simple casements with mullions. Linking the interiors to the out-of-doors is important to a camp-like atmosphere. Doors would be plank or frame and flat-paneled. Entrance doors would be heavy planks or timber, the rougher the better.

Moldings

Moldings fashioned from peeled logs or split timbers would be used, along with wide, flat boards simply worked and without adornment.

Photo courtesy of GE Appliances

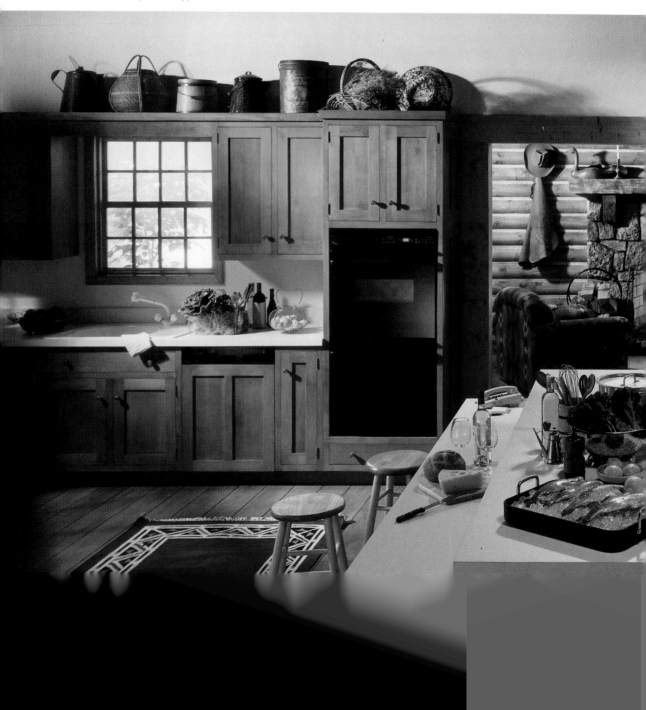

This Lodge-styled kitchen combines simple frame and panel cabinetry, wide plank floors and heavy timber beams. It opens to an exposed log-paneled room with a massive river rock fireplace and Indian blanket upholstery for a complete atmosphere of a bunkhouse or mountain lodge.

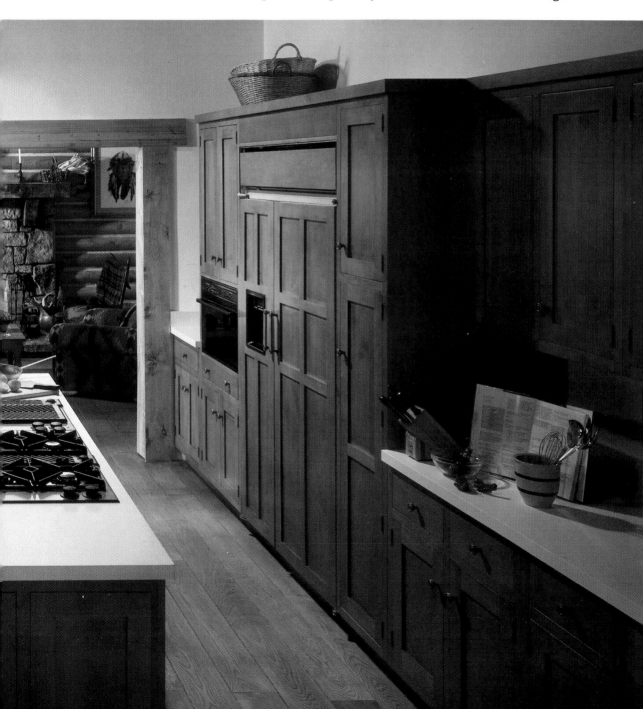

Cabinetry

Pine or oak cabinets in plank door styles or square raised or recessed panels. Decorative recessed panels could be tooled in leather, punched tin or detailed with applied twig moldings. Cherry cabinets can enhance the rich, warm hearth-side feeling, if not too grand in style.

Countertops

Countertops could be wood, slate, soapstone or tile.

Floors

Floors are generally made of flagstone or wide, random plank wood. Softer woods such as fir and pine will develop a distressed patina which is in keeping with the theme.

Rustic "twig" furniture.

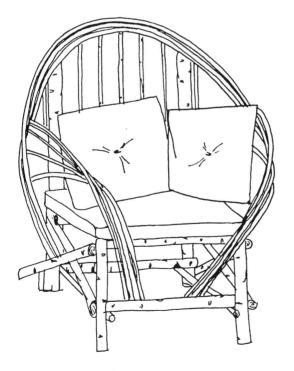

Furniture

Furnishings should have a very comfortable, lived-in look. In the same way that Queen Anne is a more relaxed version of Victorian style, Lodge style is the most rustic form of Arts and Crafts. Mismatched furnishings and the look of a leisurely lifestyle evokes memories of summer vacations at the lake and a homey, friendly atmosphere. Furniture and built-ins consist of rustic pole furnishings, local river rocks and heavy exposed timber framing.

Fabrics

Fabrics that suit this style include heavy woven blanket wools, homespun Native American designs and motifs, lightweight cotton checks and plaids for contrast and balance.

Wallcoverings

Wallcoverings would be used sparingly, in small prints or nature motifs. More typical wall treatments would be woven hangings or rugs.

Accessories

Many natural motifs are used in accessorizing: animal pelts (perhaps fake), antlers, baskets, fishing gear, saddles and tack, landscape paintings and botanical prints all add a feeling of authenticity. Terra cotta and southwest elements are suitable in the West and Southwest. This is a style that works best when strongly tied in to the local landscape.

*An **adventurous Lodge-like, yet elegant,** bathroom.*

Courtesy of Kohler Co.

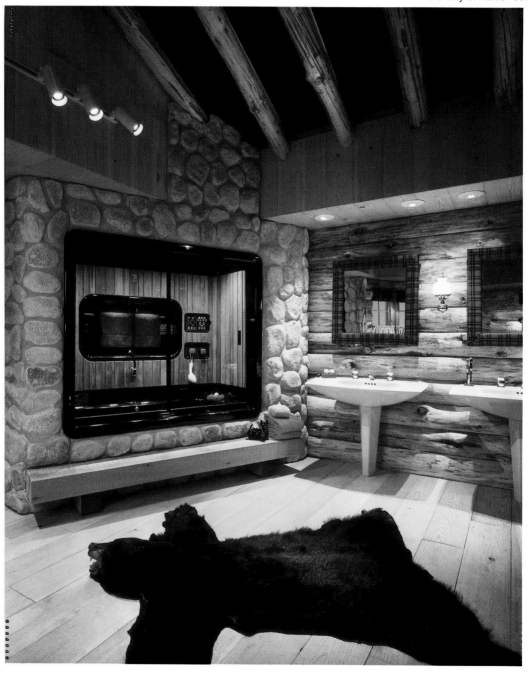

Pine plank walls and cabinetry combined with vaguely Victorian decorative elements suggest a western frontier feel to this bathroom.

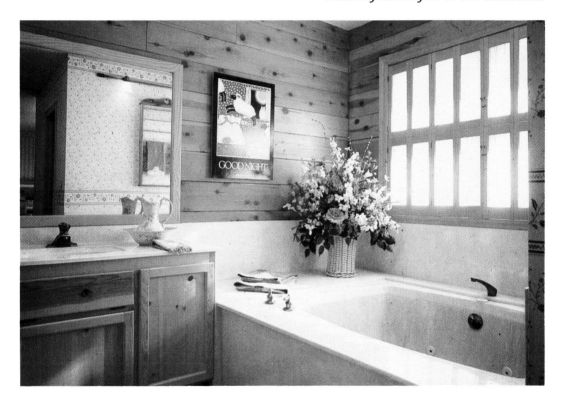

RUSTIC
Prairie School

Historic Context
The Prairie School describes a group of Chicago-area architects who based their ideas primarily on the principles and examples of Frank Lloyd Wright. An outgrowth of the Craftsman era, Wright built on the concept of the bungalow to develop housing that seemed to grow out of its surrounding landscape, with strong Midwest roots. In Wright's architecture, interior furnishings were supposed to carry out the theme of the architecture, and ultimately became an important structural element of the theme. The use of built-ins was common, and much of the Arts and Crafts styling is appropriate, too, but this style should also be a bit more sophisticated and contemporary in appearance.

Walls/Ceilings
Coffered or chamfered ceilings would be adorned with box beams or left plain and relatively low for a horizontal emphasis.

Windows/Doors
Most often grouped together in horizontal bands to emphasize and accentuate the dominance of horizontal lines in this style of architecture. Use of decorative leaded glass in geometric patterns was common.

Moldings
Moldings would be square edged, or bullnosed in crisp and clean lines. Strong horizontal lines repeat the emphasis of the architectural style.

Cabinetry
Cabinetry of very clean and simple lines demonstrate the style best. Clear fir, mahogany, rift-cut oaks, walnut, teak and cherry would all be appropriate, with recessed panel or flush overlay doors with square-edged details. European-style "over-bodens," overhead shelves that incorporate lighting, would also be effective in a Prairie kitchen, tying banks of cabinetry together. Stainless

Frank Lloyd Wright designed many leaded glass window patterns that are at once Art Nouveau, Art Deco, Native American and Craftsman in their motifs and stylization.

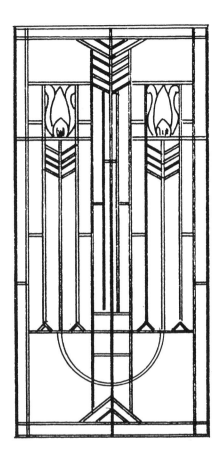

steel cabinetry would also be appropriate, as Wright stressed using suitable and practical materials for their intended use and ease of maintenance.

Countertops

Patterned ceramic tiles, granite, wood, slate, soapstone, solid-surface countertop materials, and even stainless steel, would all be suitable choices for the Prairie style.

Floors

Ceramic- or quarry-tiled floors or geometric patterned vinyls, with Native American woven rugs or cotton dhurries could be used.

Furniture

In Wright's architecture, interior furnishing carried out the theme of the architecture and was an important structural element. Many built-ins were common, and much of the Arts and Crafts styling is appropriate, but with a little more sophistication and contemporary lines. Often times, contemporary furnishings blend well in a Prairie-style house.

This Prairie-styled kitchen combines the simple lines of Craftsman cabinets with architectural pulls, Frank Lloyd Wright leaded glass, high-tech lighting and a uniquely stylized dentil molding.

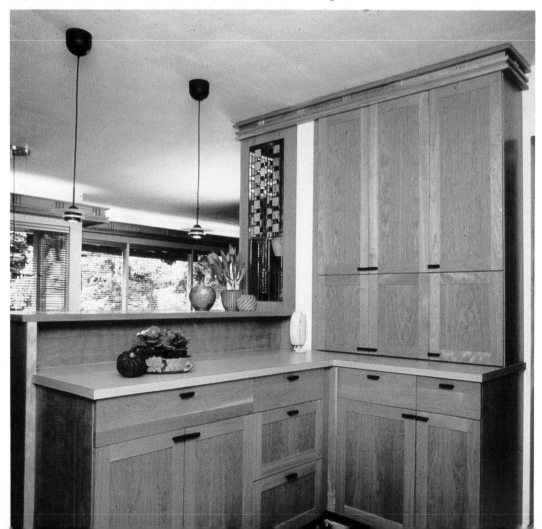

Fabrics

Prairie School fabrics would be very similar to Craftsman fabrics in that they would employ natural fibers and dyes, perhaps with more woven or geometric patterns included.

Wallcoverings

Primarily textural, but not as common as other wall surface treatments. Some wallcovering manufacturers, such as Schumacher, have revived some Frank Lloyd Wright fabric patterns and have incorporated them into wallpapers for a special collection in his honor. In a true Prairie interior, if wallcoverings were used, they would be primarily grass cloths, linens or rice paper.

Accessories

Many of the same accessories that work in a Craftsman style translate well to this look. However, spare, structural design is best, not overly decorated or accessorized. Chrome fittings and spare use of glass block might be used.

RUSTIC
Mission
(Spanish Mission Revival)

Historic Context
This style features many Mediterranean influences, particularly Spanish and Moorish, however, classical elements of ancient history and religious imagery are also incorporated. Most often found in warmer climates, houses in the hacienda style work best when open to the outdoors. It is interesting to note that the early California ranchos are believed to be the prototypes for the U-shaped ranch house that is designed around a central patio.

Walls/Ceilings
Adobe, rough plaster in rustic pale tones contrasting with heavy, dark exposed ceiling beams in vaulted or flat ceilings, was used. Off-white walls with pale fresco color tints are most common. Tile wainscots were typically found in bathrooms. Fireplaces are a dominant focal point of the room, often plastered, with tile trim and hearths.

Windows/Doors
Wooden shutters at the windows, trimmed with wrought iron grills at the exteriors, were often used.

Moldings
Doors and windows were trimmed with heavily carved, dark woods or sometimes trimmed out in ceramic tile or plaster wrapped.

Cabinetry
Oak or pine might be used and sometimes walnut, with heavy, raised panel or board and batten solid-wood door styles. Finishes would be rich, darker stains, or limed (white washed).

Countertops
Glazed ceramic tile adds rich color; butcher-block or natural stone counters would also work well.

Rustic pine cabinetry and solid-surface countertops resembling stone combine with the plaster hood, American Indian motif backsplash tile and verdigris metal accents for a weathered southwestern version of Mission Revival.

Designed by Lynn Wallace, CKD; Courtesy of Fry Communications

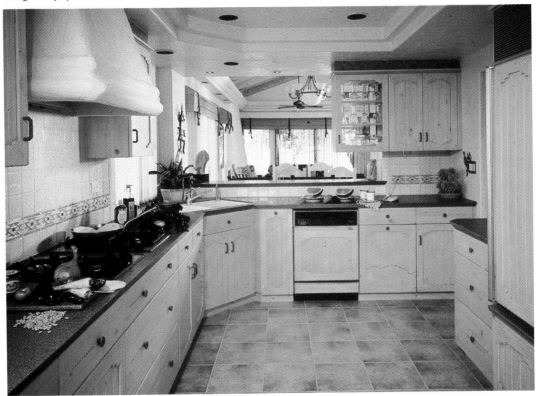

Terra-cotta pavers are artfully combined with glazed teal tile in this Spanish Mission Revival bathroom. Off-white plastered walls, wide blade shutters and the arched shape of the decorative glass panels softly fill in the background. The etched cactus and moon patterns are both whimsical and evocative of the southwestern desert.

Designed by Margie Little, CKD and Dianne Hynes; Photo by David Livingston

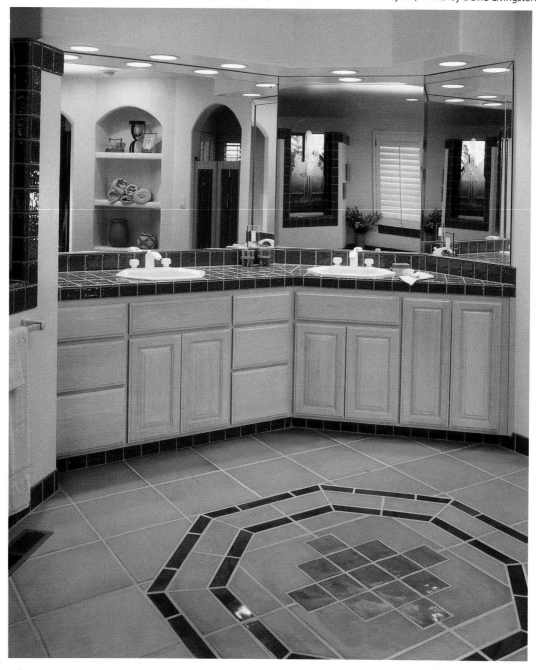

Designed by Margie Little, CKD and Dianne Hynes; Photo by David Livingston

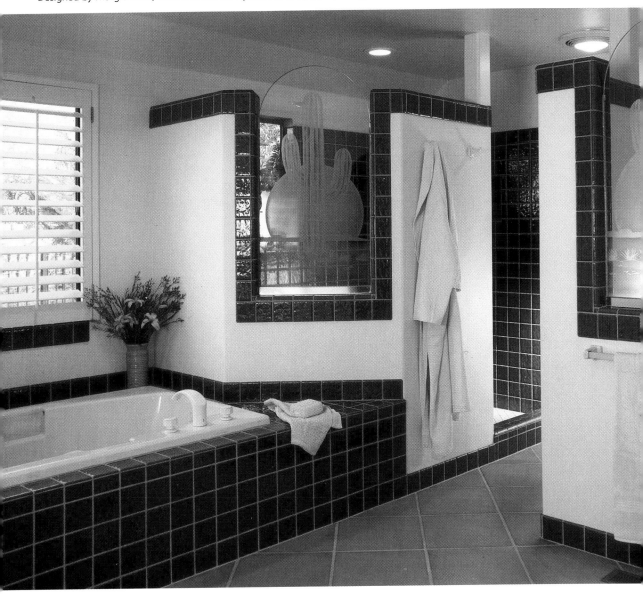

Floors

Tile or wood floors, brick or rustic pavers would be most typical. Floors would be wide random-plank oak, terra cotta paver tiles, colorfully glazed ceramic tiles covered with American Indian rugs or woven dhurries, with some geometric patterned Oriental carpets as well. In the bathroom, glazed ceramic tiles would be carried up the walls.

Furniture

Straight-legged Mission pieces would be typical, also Jacobean turned-legged chairs and tables and styles similar to Tudor Revival pieces, using dark oak, Spanish mahogany, woven leather strap seats and benches, pale limed woods with some gold leaf and silver accents.

The rustic glazed tile, arched doorway niche and rough-textured plaster walls are all elements that combine to make an effective Spanish Mission Revival look.

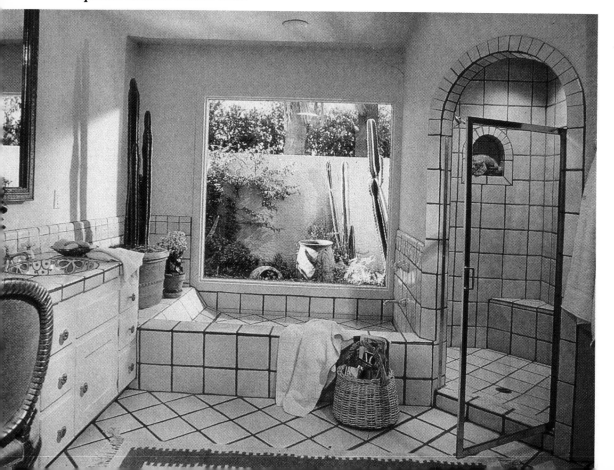

Fabrics

Silk, woven tapestries and natural fibers work best. Colors would include pale pink, subtle grays, terra cotta, verdigris, silver, rust and dark browns.

Wallcoverings

Tapestry wall hangings would typically adorn plain heavy plaster walls.

Accessories

Appropriate accessory choices include vellum or parchment shades on lamps, which may be hand painted, Native American pottery and baskets, ferns, cactus, "structural"-looking large plants, which link the inside to the outside, and wrought iron.

Tile floors, countertops and range hood are mixed with lime-washed cabinetry and plaster detailing in this Spanish Mission or Santa Fe-themed kitchen.

Photo courtesy of Fry Communications

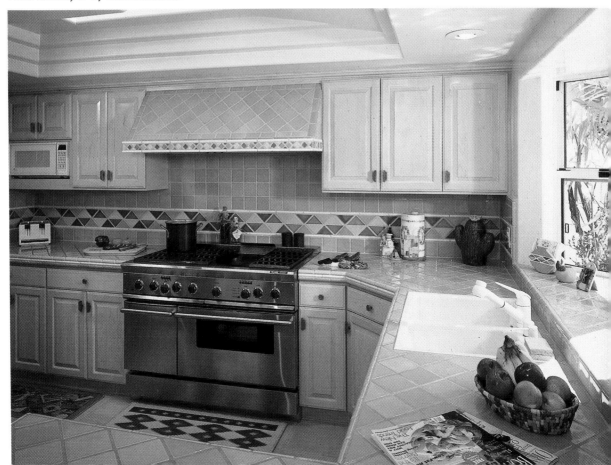

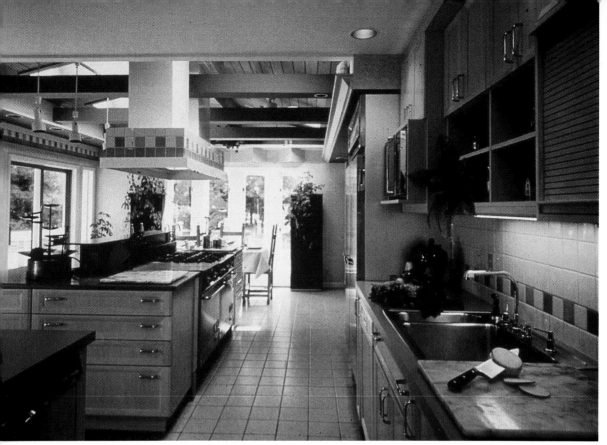

Designed by Alice Harold; Photo courtesy of Fry Communications

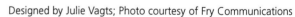

Designed by Julie Vagts; Photo courtesy of Fry Communications

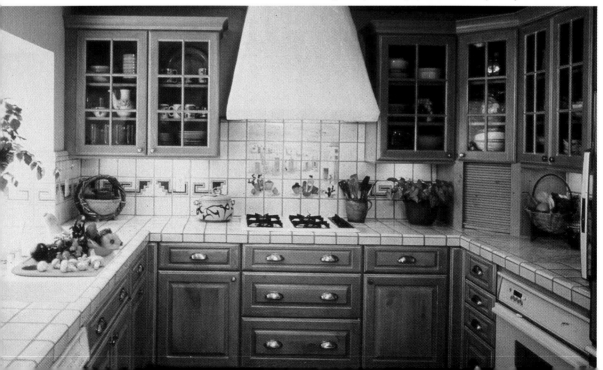

REVIVAL
Tudor Revival

Historic Context
This style actually has some spillover into Arts and Crafts and English Country. Loosely based on medieval English prototypes ranging from thatch-roofed cottages to grand manor houses, it is a style that freely mixes materials and themes. The more modest cottage Tudor Revival look was very popular in the 1920s. Tudor

Parquet hardwood flooring is a typical material for all of the Baronial styles, with the possible exception of Spanish Mission, where wide-planked oak floors would be more common.

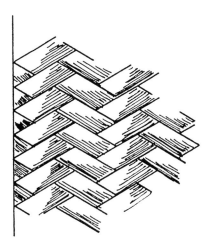

Revival interiors are infused with a spirit of adventure and exploration, and maps, globes and books frequently are used to add a scholarly air.

Walls/Ceilings
Walls are often paneled, but rustic plaster with cross timbering is also common. Plastered walls can have stenciled details or papered friezes. Ornamental stonework is also frequently used in

Rose-toned plaster walls, stylized arches adorning the cabinetry, diamond paned window, stone floor and wrought iron accessories are all elements that combine to achieve a unique interpretation of Tudor Revival style. The unfitted look gives the kitchen a cottage-like feel, which is in keeping with the spirit of Tudor Revival.

Photo courtesy of GE Appliances

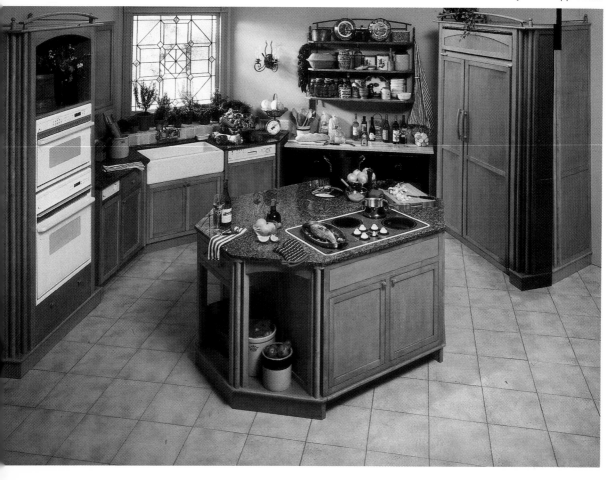

Tudor arches on doors, windows and fireplaces. Colors of raw sienna, raw umber, cream, white, parchment, slate, lead gray, deep blues and vibrant yellow are all suitable.

Windows/Doors
Windows were often leaded in diamond-patterned panes. Lancet arches on focal windows add to the theme. Treatment is typically velvet, tapestry or woven draperies in simple styling, hung from wrought-iron rods.

Moldings
Much the same as the Baronial styles, incorporating Gothic tracery and gingerbread trellis work, executed in wood, iron or plaster. Sometimes moldings on walls would be built-up out of plaster and highlighted with warm white, cream or pastel paint tones.

Cabinetry
Dark, antique or lime-washed oak in frame, raised or recessed panel door styles, incorporating a lancet arch, if possible. Leaded, clear glass inserts in diamond patterns would be appropriate to detail this look. While earlier Gothic styles would almost exclusively be limited to oak, Tudor Revival cabinetry could be fashioned out of oak, mahogany, cherry, beech or any of the woods popular in the '20s.

Countertops
Laminates or solid-surface materials in patterns and colors resembling slate, limestone, marble or wood can be used effectively, as well as granite, and real stone materials. Rustic glazed tiles, incorporating heraldic motifs, would also be appropriate.

Floors
Wide-planked woods in dark tones or lime-washed oak, brick or stone would be typical.

Furniture

Furnishings would feature the heavy, straight lines of the Mission-type furniture, but carved, Jacobean twisted-leg forms would also be present. Tables with arched stretchers, and ball foot and claw foot details are all suitable. Oak is the most typical wood choice. This style has much spillover into Arts and Crafts, English Country and Baronial styles. Loosely based on medieval English prototypes ranging from thatched roofed cottages to grand manor houses, it is a style of freely mixed materials and themes. The more modest Tudor Revival look was very popular in the 1920s.

Fabrics

Fabrics associated with the style include leather and heavy tapestries similar to the Baronial style, but with the added cottage-like chintzes, homespuns and printed linens. Florals tend to be stylized natural forms and toile-type pastoral scenes on white or cream backgrounds.

Wallcoverings

Similar to the Baronial style, gilt, gold and silver leaf detailing, heraldic motifs, small, open patterns or gothic trelliswork were used. Tudor Revival also incorporates use of rich detail resembling tapestries, toiles, stylized florals and woven textures. Mythical, magical and exotic themes are also appropriate.

Accessories

Tudor Revival interiors are infused with a spirit of adventure and exploration. Maps, globes and books add a scholarly air. Other accessories include pewter, brass, copper, tooled leather and fine ceramic pottery.

MODERN
Art Deco and Savoy

Historic Context

Styles of ornaments that were especially popular in the '20s and '30s, Art Deco and Savoy are readily identified by their frets, zigzags, chevrons and angular, stylized floral motifs. Occurring during a period of pronounced poverty, these styles are associated with a special kind of sophistication, which revolved around taking chaste, classical forms and reworking them to the point of nearly absolute reduction and minimalism. Savoy style, which refers to the more distinctly luxurious interpretations of Art Deco style, was named after the famous grand hotel in London, conjuring up images of luxurious penthouse suites and glamorous interpretations of Hollywood film sets.

Walls/Ceilings

Walls were generally adorned with complex-patterned friezes, accented in brass or gold leaf and decorative bronze and aluminum panels. Abstract geometrical designs predominated,

Deco-styled furniture employed exotic veneers to achieve the smooth, curved shapes for which the style is noted.

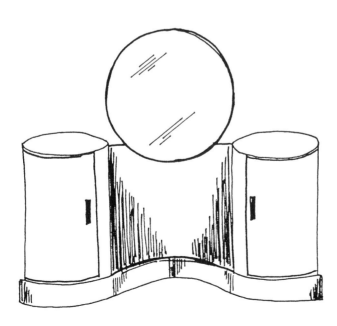

with Aztec and Mayan patterns used, as well as classical motifs and Egyptian imagery. Colors of red, green, bronze, silver and pink, lemon and turquoise, cream and beige background tones with black accents, muddy mustards to lemon yellow, mint green, blue and candy pink were used. Warmer tones of peach, apricot, yellow and pale cream were also popular.

Windows/Doors
Portholes and glass block used as architectural detail was noteworthy in this style. Period casement windows were often metal framed, with horizontal mullions.

Moldings
Moldings were pronounced, but in streamlined forms. Stairstepped "ziggurat" style moldings were often employed to add drama and depth to a room and to cabinetry.

Cabinetry
Cabinetry featured clean lines incorporating curves in dark or pale washed finishes with decorative metal accents. Glossy or painted enameled finishes are also appropriate. The Savoy styles tend to have more elegant detailing, whereas Deco styling is more austere and streamlined. Smooth, flush door styles are most common.

Countertops
Marble, sleek soapstone, granite and laminates would be most complimentary to this style. Tiles laid in either high contrast or colorful geometric patterns would also work well.

Floors
Mosaic tile floors, marble tile and elegant parquet patterns with intricate inlays were all featured. Carpets tended to be geometric and abstract in design.

Furniture

Furniture and woodwork were often fashioned out of exotic wood veneers of beautifully figured woods. Furnishings were frequently ornamented with inlays of brightly colored lacquers, other woods and ebony. Decorative motifs of stylized trees, shells, fans and sunrises were all typical. Furniture had rounded outlines and often was adorned with exotic materials, such as ivory and snakeskin. The introduction of the cocktail cabinet and the coffee table came about during this era.

Fabrics

Ethereal silks, chiffons and satins combined with the sumptuous texture of heavy, fake fur would be evocative of the Savoy style, while a sparer Deco setting would incorporate more woven textures and geometric patterns. Leather, fur and metallic wovens all combine to add interest and texture to this look.

Wallcoverings

Gold and silver leafing, painted finishes suggesting texture, stripes and geometric patterns and simplified Art Nouveau motifs would contribute to the effect.

Accessories

Oriental elements such as Chinese vases, pagoda lamp shades, mandarins and dragons were combined with unlikely items such as glass block, chrome and frosted Lalique glass.

MODERN
International

Historic Context

Rooted in the famous German school of design called the Bauhaus, which was founded in 1919, the International style gave design a new and pure direction, idealizing industrialization. Although the school, with its new architecture, was closed by Hitler in 1933, the people and the ideas of the Bauhaus migrated throughout the world: hence the name, International. The essence of the modern movement comes from its dogmatism. From 1900 to 1930, the design world was guided by such names and phrases as:

"*Form follows function.*" - Walter Gropius
"*Less is more.*" - Mies Van der Rohe
"*A house is a machine to live in.*" - Le Corbusier

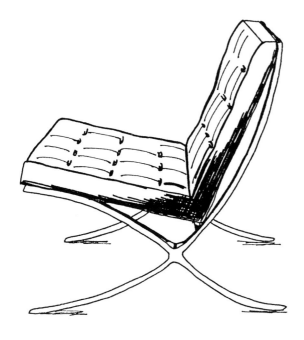

International architects often designed furniture to fit their meticulously simple designs.

The architectural philosophy of modernism was based on aesthetic relationships and pure geometric form. The same ideals are seen in Cubist painting and sculpture of the time. The idea was that the architect could effect social change by designing buildings which rejected gaudy ornamentation, focusing instead on functionality and simplicity. In accordance with this philosophy, buildings were designed in basic units and were constructed and furnished in "honest" materials—glass, concrete and steel. Flat roofs and walls of glass showed a pronounced lack of color and detail.

An International-styled kitchen would utilize materials for their practicality and function. Here, the stainless steel on the wall cabinets and countertops is celebrated for its nature of durability and strength. Form and line are reduced to their essence.

Designed by Gay Fly, CKD, CBD

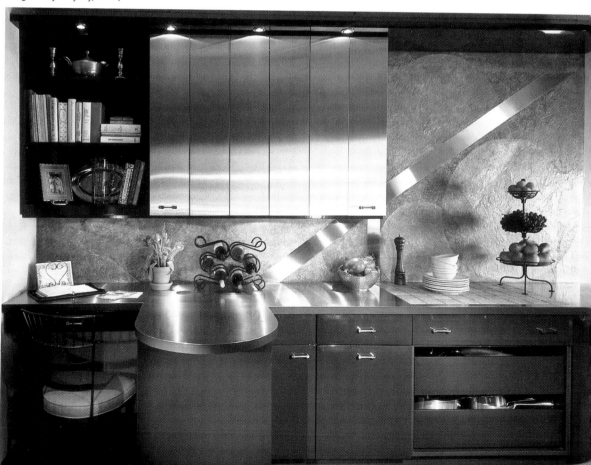

Walls/Ceilings

Subtle color palettes and variety of texture play against spare, monochromatic architectural space.

Windows/Doors

Buildings were designed in basic units, and were constructed and furnished in "honest" materials—glass, concrete, steel. Flat roofs and walls of glass were remarkable for their lack of color and detail.

Moldings

Door and window casings were minimal or absent altogether.

Cabinetry

To develop an International style in the kitchen, it is necessary to first understand the basics of modern design. Functionalism and the absence of applied ornamentation are at the heart of every successful modern theme. The intrinsic beauty of texture in a material, which lends itself to the purpose and form of that object, is basic to modern design. Cabinetry of simple flush overlay design, crafted in rich veneers, stainless steel or crisp laminates would contribute successfully to the theme. Cabinets and fixtures would be arranged architecturally, creating a form out of the space they occupy.

Countertops

The richly translucent matte finish of a synthetic solid surface or a granite countertop are attractive and perform well as countertop material selections in this style.

Floors

Flooring could be slate, light-colored stone, polished cement or wood, covered with American Indian woven carpets or flat woven dhurrie rugs. In the kitchens or bathrooms, linoleum that looks like linoleum (not stone, tile or wood prints) would be suitable.

Furniture

Furnishings of contemporary lines, often designed by architects, reflect the inspiration of both the Biedermeier and Empire styles—sleek, spare and of simplified classical inspiration.

Fabrics

Any material or color combination is appropriate, as long as it is an honest presentation and devoid of unnecessary decoration and ornamentation.

The simplicity and accessibility designed into this bathroom epitomizes the concepts of International design.

Designed by Ingrid Becker, CKD; Courtesy of Decorating & Remodeling Magazine

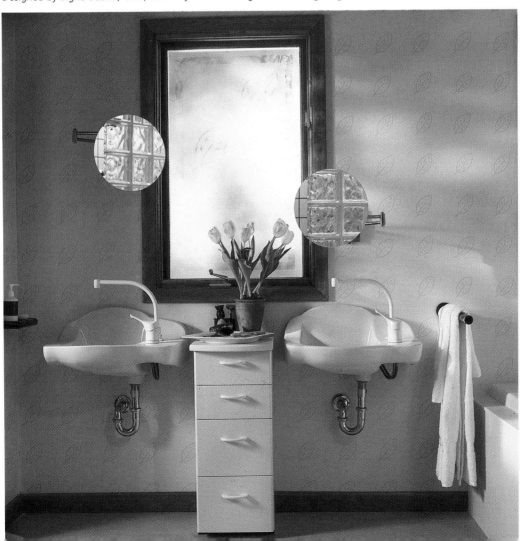

Wallcoverings

Wallcoverings were typically not present; an International modernist would disdain any faux finishes or look-alike products.

Accessories

Accessories would be large scale, sculptural and used very sparingly. Dramatic use of flowers and plants would be appropriate, if not overdone.

A serene and simple bathroom combines form and function to create timeless beauty. The skillful use of both natural and synthetic light give this bathroom an ethereal "other world" feel.

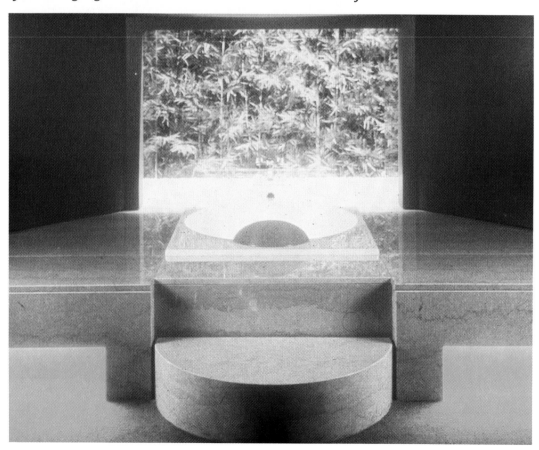

Courtesy of Subzero Co.

Everything in this wet bar is designed for utmost function and convenience.

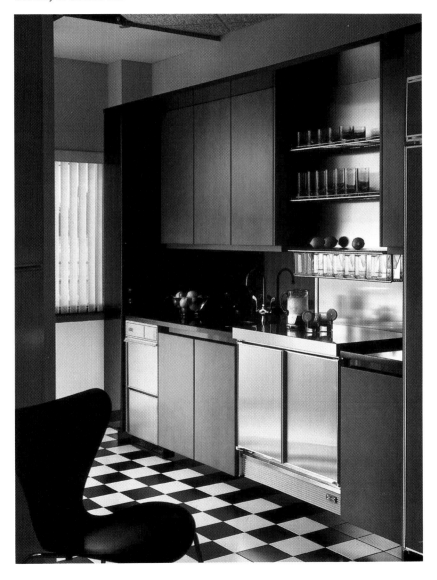

COUNTRY

The various and enduringly popular Country styles reflect a basic celebration of the countryside, and are based on certain fundamental components—natural materials and colors, functional design, good craftsmanship, homespun skills and the relationship of the indoors to the outdoors, which is often forgotten in contemporary urban life.

The country styles focus primarily on interior style, and can occur in Georgian- and Colonial-style homes, from humble cottages to grand manor houses. Typically more suited to the traditional building styles, any of the Country styles (with the exception of Contemporary International styles) can be effectively employed in most architectural styles, especially in the kitchen and bathroom, which are considered the realm of the family, and therefore less formal than other parts of the house.

Country style is one of simplicity and practicality, borne out of a response to local climate and landscape. The focus is on honest use of materials, ingenious resourcefulness, a sense of tradition and a reliance on local materials.

Here we will discuss four of the most popular Country styles: French Country, American Country, English Country and Swedish Country. There are, of course, as many Country looks as there are countries. Some of the others that are gaining in popularity are Italian, Irish and Tropical (Plantation Style) Country.

COUNTRY
French Country

Historic Context
French Country is attributed to a style invented by prosperous farmers, originally copying Parisian court styles, interpreting the sophisticated and pretentious motifs with skilled workmanship, ingenuity and delightful naiveté. A study in unpretentiousness, a Country French kitchen or bathroom would house a variety of mismatched patterns, colors and textures.

Walls/Ceilings
Walls of distressed, heavy plaster, perhaps with some stenciling, or a combination of wallpaper colors and patterns, with heavily beamed ceilings as a counterpoint are typical. An open fireplace in the kitchen or bathroom would be ideal, if space permitted, and would add a cozy *cottage-y* feeling. Pastel colors with an introduction of more vibrant accents is common. Blue, gray, pink, peach and teal are popular, with mustard yellow, red and green accents.

Windows/Doors
Authentic French ceilings are typically higher and the windows are taller than the proportions to which we are accustomed. Existing structure may limit us, but window treatments and elaborate cornice moldings can be employed to enhance a taller look and feel.

Moldings
Classically styled and heavily carved moldings are of great importance to the look. Moldings at doors and windows should be rustic interpretations of the classical Georgian and Empire (French) styling. Usually painted, they could be dragged or crackle finished to simulate great age and countless coats of paint. Limed and whitewashed finishes are typical.

*The garden is brought inside and seems to be vining
around the fixtures in this French Country bathroom.*

Courtesy of Kohler Co.

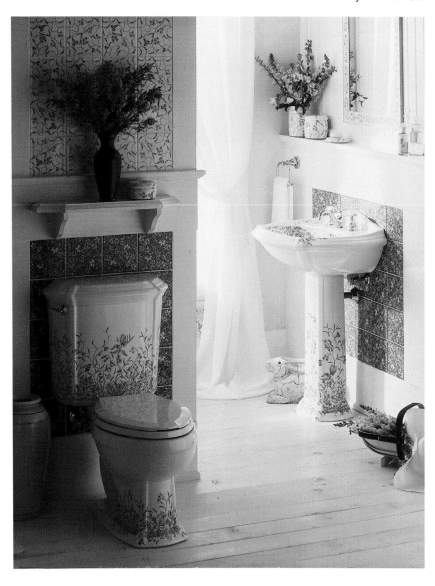

Cabinetry

In the best Country French kitchens and bathrooms, nothing would appear to be new or fixed in place. Rather, an unfitted look works best, lending a timeless informality to the setting. Cabinet doors may have arched raised panels and carved moldings to imitate the armoires and buffets of the period. Walnut, chestnut, oak, pine, cherry and fruitwoods are all appropriate, often white washed or limed for an aged look. Painted woodwork in whites, creams or pale blues would also be typical. Hardware is an important detail, with long barrel hinges the size of the doors and beautiful, fanciful hand-wrought strap hinges and pulls in brass, iron or pewter finishes.

Countertops

Wooden, tiled, marbled or granite countertops are suitable and durable. Solid surfacing and ceramic tile are also good choices. Ceramic tiles in patterns inspired by French faience in blues and white can be used in backsplashes to provide old world charm and rich color. Solid surface counters may feature intricate inlays or gently sculpted edge details.

Floors

Floors were often wood, limestone or paved, with rough terra cotta quarry tiles. Hardwood floors were parquet or plank. Ceramic tiles, flagstone or even marble in a rustic, worn state would be appropriate.

Furniture

French cabinet making was a highly prized skill, and good pieces of furniture were designed to last for centuries and were considered a worthy investment to be handed down for generations. The grand armoires and buffets of the period were focal points and grand beyond their humble surroundings. These pieces were often part of a young woman's dowry and a symbol of a family's wealth. The carvings on detachable crowns often featured love birds symbolizing fidelity, grain baskets symbolizing prosperity, and vine leaves for long life. Typical materials used were oak, elm, walnut, pearwood and cherry. Furnishings would usually incorporate curved, feminine lines. Eclectic and cozy, the occasional grand piece or authentic antique can establish the sense of a French Country theme and serve as a focal point from which to build. Everything should look as if it were gathered over time. Large French Country harvest tables would often dominate a kitchen. Designed as a work surface, their deep, carved aprons and drawers prohibit drawing a chair up to them.

Designed by Tess Giuliani, CKD; Photo by Harriett Weiss

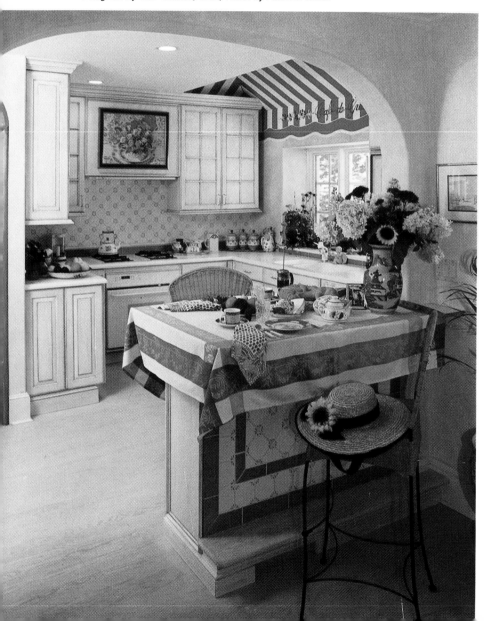

Blue and white motif, a garden-like atmosphere and a tromp l'oeil awning give one the sense of a sidewalk cafe in this French Country kitchen.

Fabrics

Fabrics were rough, nubby woven wools and wonderfully colorful wood block printed cottons, made popular by the importer Pierre Deux. These were mixed with fancy French damasks, silks, brocades and jacquards. Small print or checked chintzes may complement a grander scaled floral or glazed chintz, damask or toile de jouy, a French print that features delicately rendered images of pastoral scenes, usually in one color on a white or cream background. Toiles tend to give a room a more formal feel.

Carved arched valances add furniture-like detail in Country French design. The floral theme of the mural establishes the needed link to the garden essential to a successful Country look.

Designed by Ellen Cheever, ASID, CBD, CKD; Photo courtesy of Kohler Co.

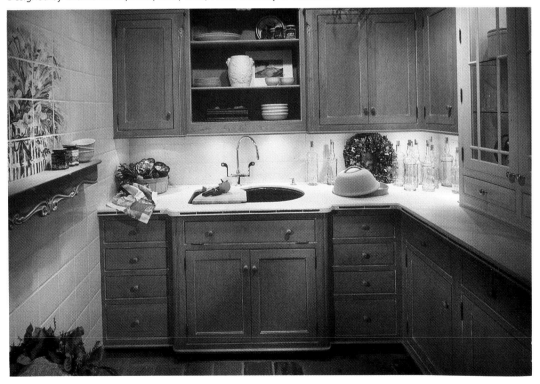

Wallcoverings

Wallcoverings would be abundantly present in all the colors and textures of the fabrics typical to the style.

Accessories

Accessories of copper, baskets and locally produced crockery in terra cotta or brightly colored Quimper ware (pronounced "campair") add richness of detail. Many varieties of painted porcelains, called faience, as well as pewter and silver are typical. Lace adorns windows and dresses up open shelves.

Lime-washed and aged finishes on the cabinets enhance the aged rustic and antique feel of a Country French kitchen. The commercial range is an eloquent focal point, adorned with a molded plaster hood. Lace, flowers and luscious fruits bring the countryside indoors.

Courtesy of Wm Ohs Exquisite Handmade Kitchens

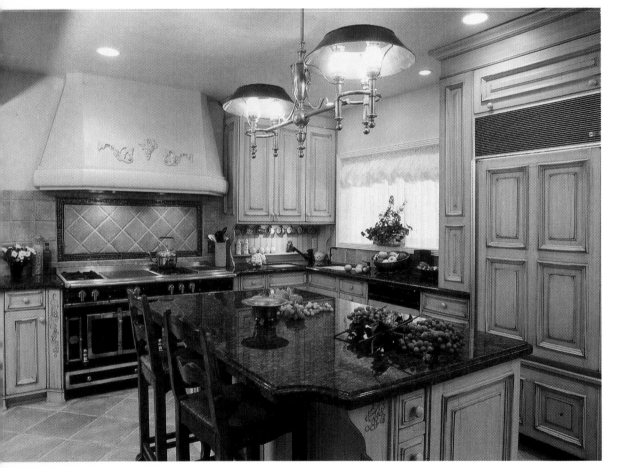

COUNTRY
English Country

Historic Context

From small and quaint cottage settings to grand country manor houses, the English preference for Georgian and Gothic schemes defines the major differences of English Country and French Country. The principles of rustic interpretations of Georgian court style with elements of Gothic heraldry were generally followed.

Walls/Ceilings

Plaster, with half-timbering present, brick infill or wallpapered with flowery chintz prints, Gothic and Arts and Crafts motifs work as well.

Windows/Doors

Much the same as would be found in Classical or Baronial styles, with Palladian arched or Lancet arched focal windows and doorways. Interior doors could be frame and raised panels or planked.

Moldings

Heavy, complex Georgian and Tudor style moldings work well, in white or cream painted finishes, or limed, dragged or crackled to give a rustic texture and worn, aged look.

Cabinetry

Oak, pine, cherry or walnut cabinets in square raised or recessed panels add rich warmth, but painted gleaming woodwork is also quite typical. Beaded inset doors or heavily applied moldings also work well. Beaded board interiors or paneling, open dish racks and fretwork are typical details.

Countertops

Countertops of any available surface work well in an English Country kitchen, with fairly simple edge detailing.

Floors

Brick, wood plank or parquet, limestone pavers and stone.

The Aga range is the quintessential English Country element. In this kitchen, it is artfully blended into the rich bead boarding and cabinet fretwork. Open shelves and glazed cabinet doors relieve an otherwise massive wall of cabinetry. The open hutch adds an unfitted furniture look to the room. Rustic pavers on the floor enhance a country feel.

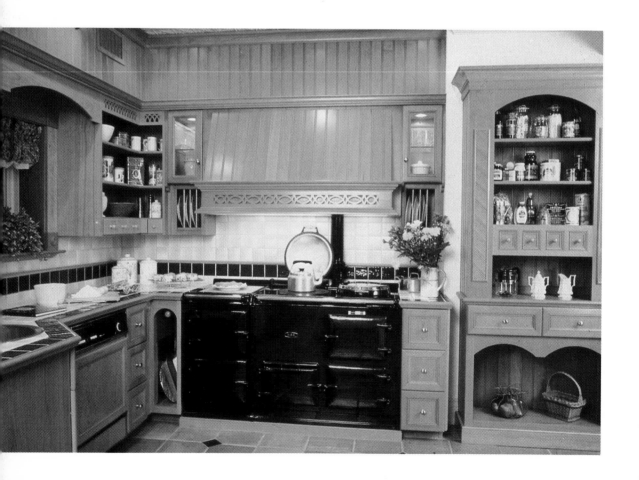

This English Country kitchen is of the grand manor genre. The commercial-styled cooking equipment, soapstone countertops, fretwork, grand-scaled moldings and heroic pot rack all support the theme.

Designed by Thomas Kling, CKD

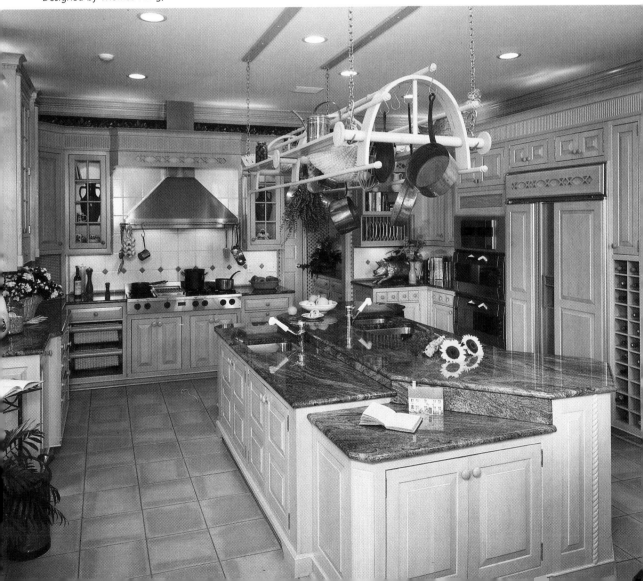

Furniture

Pieces from Queen Anne, Gothic and Georgian styles can all blend in jumbled harmony. Old Welsh dressers (buffets with open shelves above) display pewter, Dresden, Canton and Spode china—the more the merrier.

Fabrics

Fabrics are blended together like a wild cottage garden, with glazed cotton chintz, rich with colors and cabbage roses, as the mainstay. Small scale Liberty prints fill in and textural wovens and Nottingham lace blend happily together to create a pleasant, homey and informal atmosphere.

Wallcoverings

Small prints or large scale florals, stripes or all three combined are common types of wallcoverings. Nothing too refined or formal, but informality and coziness are the desired feelings to be achieved in all wallcovering applications and combinations.

Accessories

Copper, brass, pewter, baskets, Oriental china and teapots, lace and linens, and flowers everywhere fill an English Country interior scheme. The most successful interiors have strong links to the outdoors and the countryside.

In this view, the pine armoire and country-styled gingham prints help to "informalize" the more casual areas of the room.

Designed by Thomas Kling, CKD

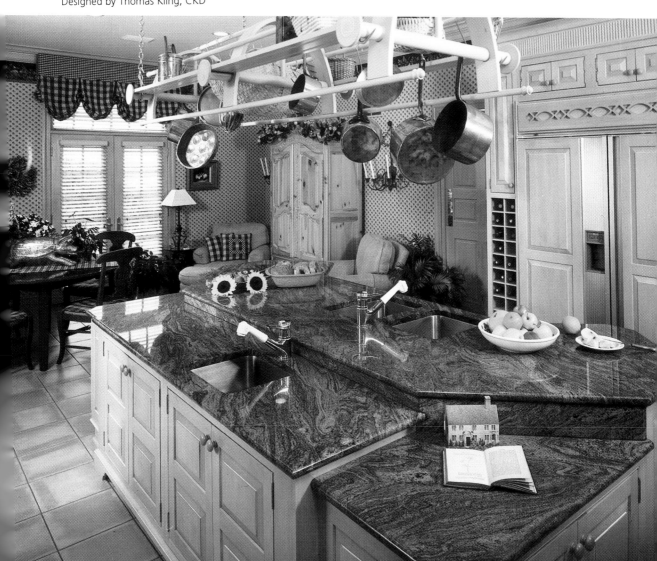

COUNTRY
American Country

Historic Context

American Country style draws heavily from American Colonial influences, but local regional vintage themes are well blended in with them. For example, the popular Cowboy style is effectively employed in the West and Southwestern regions, while true Colonial styles tend to be more commonly used in the New England states. The Midwest and Prairie states tend to employ a Farmhouse Country theme in the homes of that region. Simplicity and practicality are the hallmarks of American Country style. Turned wood posts, straight lines and square shapes define sturdy, sometimes primitively crafted elements.

Walls/Ceilings

Walls would be rough plaster, painted white or off white, with milk painted or natural finished woodwork trim. Flat board paneling, bead board paneling or simple wainscot paneling would be typical, with stencil painted motifs or wallpaper above in rustic, unsophisticated prints. Again, regional influences and sub-themes are appropriate patterns to include.

Windows/Doors

Window treatments could feature shutters, simple cotton print or muslin casements, or rolling shades.

Moldings

Molding profiles, finishes and uses for doors, windows and baseboards are much the same as found in typical Colonial interiors. If painted, they should be finished in dull, velvety sheens.

Cabinetry

Cabinetry could be oak, pine, maple or painted in a milky finish. Cabinetry and woodwork could have a pickled or dragged finish to suggest age and many layers of paint. Color should be used

Two tones of cherry and simple, spare styling highlight the Craftsmanship that was so highly prized by the Shakers. The quilt-like pattern of the backsplash tile, baskets, herbs and an alphabet frieze complete the theme in this American Country Shaker kitchen.

Designed by Melanie Taylor, Architect and Paul Weidman, CKD; Courtesy of Decorating & Remodeling Magazine

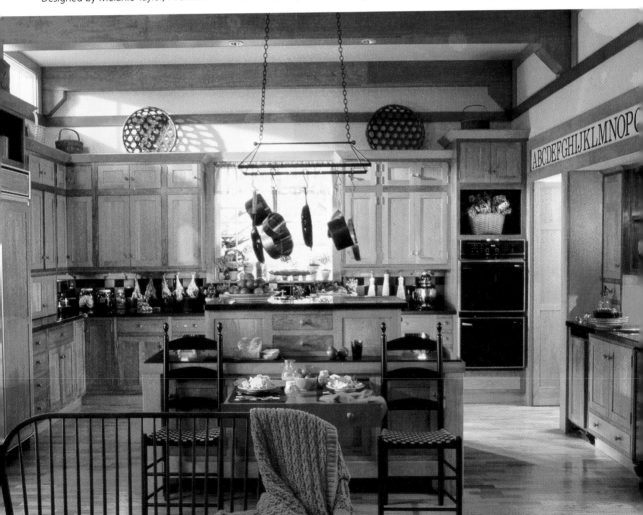

without timidness. Butted boards or stile and rail with flat panels would be the best door styles to use, generally with very simple edge details.

Countertops

Countertops could be tile, solid surface materials with very simple edge details, laminates that imitate natural stone textures and colors, granite or marble. Butcher-block would also be suitable, the more distressed in finish, the better. Wrought iron, copper, oil rubbed bronze and antiqued brass hardware and trim would work well, with visible, decorative strap hinges. Cabinetry arranged in an unfitted, furniture look will lend an old world feel to any American Country kitchen.

Floors

Maple, pine or oak planks of random widths, brick or slate, or rustic regional tile are common floor materials. Cork floors in some regions are both appropriate and practical.

Furniture

Furnishings can be eclectic and loosely assembled. An antique pine farm table and an odd assembly of press-back chairs can establish a vintage presence in a kitchen that can serve as a focal point and gathering spot. American antique hutches, pie safes and other kitchen furniture are obvious candidates, but even an antique dresser or day bed can be appropriate as well as useful in an American Country kitchen or bathroom. Any type of regional hand-crafted furnishings are typical of this look.

Fabrics

Homespuns and linens, woven wools and heavy damasks, as well as light cotton checks, plaids and chintzes, can be haphazardly blended to create an unpretentious, homey feel. Strong use of primary colors (reds, blues and yellows) is encouraged. Also, greens ranging from pale mints to rich forest greens are appropriate and can complement warm wood tones effectively.

Reds range from deep iodine and maroons to pale salmons and peaches. Yellow golds are a typical American Country color, but they are suffering from their overexposure in the "harvest gold" era, and are not as popular, but should not be ignored or avoided in any American Country scheme.

Wallcoverings

Wallcovering patterns and colors are much the same as fabrics typical to the style. Textures, small prints, checks and plaids are the most frequently used.

Accessories

Accessories of copper, iron, basketry, pottery and any handmade, traditional wares fit the style. Woven rugs from American Indian to braided rag rugs or flat woven dhurries all work well. Wood stoves and antique looking appliances are often incorporated effectively.

This version of American Country style has strong ties to the environment of a Cape Cod fishing village, in which we would expect it to be located.

Courtesy of Amana Appliances

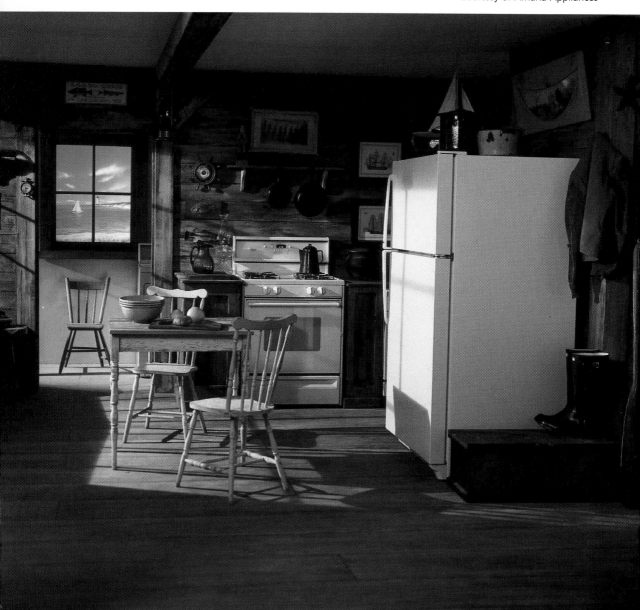

COUNTRY
Swedish Country

Historic Context

Swedish Country style, like French, English and American Country styles, generally is a more rustic and innocent interpretation of the royal court styles of the aristocratic classes. In Sweden, historic periods of political and economic strength were out-shadowed by longer periods of decline, resulting in a more unique and inventive interpretation of European fashions. Available materials were used instead of costly and rare ones. As Sweden is a heavily forested country, softwoods were most plentiful, followed by linen, wool, then, with increasing industrialization and foreign trade, glass, cotton and ceramics. Swedish style is loosely broken down into four main periods: Baroque; the French influenced Rococo; Swedish Neoclassical, or Gustavian; and Arts and Crafts, made popular in intellectual circles by the artist Carl Larsson. Larsson and his wife, Karin, decorated their family oriented country home in a uniquely Swedish interpretation of the eclectic decorative style and immortalized it in a book of his paintings, entitled A Home. This charming pictorial record of their large family's day-to-day life in this wonderful country home serves as a guide to the essence of Swedish Country Style.

Walls/Ceilings

Wood paneled walls were more common than costly plaster and were most often painted or limewashed. Walls are generally painted in soft, pastel shades. Often, they are brightened with spattering, stenciling and faux painting effects.

Windows/Doors

Sunshine and light are treasured commodities in a country with such long, dark winters, and windows were typically left untreated or shaded by very plain blinds or simple curtains made of cotton or muslin. Mirrors are placed to enhance the sun's effects. Doorways between rooms were usually left open, creating visual links between rooms and an open floor plan effect.

Moldings

Window and door trims were usually painted and sometimes faux-painted to mimic more costly materials. Architectural features and carvings on moldings were often faked with painted treatments. Chair rails and dado panels were simply painted onto flat walls, and moldings were worked in gray and white highlights to appear elaborately carved.

Cabinetry

The uncluttered look is an important hallmark of the Swedish Country style, and storage is an important element. Ample storage in sideboards or dressers and cupboards would be desirable. Open shelving in the kitchen is also common, with the contents arranged in an orderly and symmetrical fashion. Painted or pale lime washed finishes are common, with rustic faux finishes such as spattering, which was often confined to the interior of the cabinet for a whimsical touch. Pine and spruce would be the primary woods used. Simple frame and recessed panel doorstyles with delicate, applied moldings in the Gustavian and classical motifs would be common. Corner cabinets, sometimes with rounded fronts, are typical of the look.

Countertops

Wooden countertops would be most typical, but wood printed laminates, or rustic stone and ceramic tile would also be appropriate.

Floors

Wooden floors were either scrubbed and left bare, lime washed, or painted white or silver-gray to reflect the light. In grander homes, the pine floors would be faux-painted to resemble costlier woods or even marble. Rag rugs made from old clothes added a splash of color. Unique to Swedish style, long, narrow, woven runners were laid as strips running around the edges of a room and folded into miters at the corners. Traditional Gustavian colors would be stripes or checks in red, gray, cream or pale blue.

Furniture

Country Swedish furnishings are kept plain and designed to be moved around as needed. Most furniture is made out of native pine or spruce. Painted finishes are commonly employed to make them appear more sophisticated and refined. Gustavian furniture was more simple and austere than the French Neoclassic, with pale yellow details instead of gold and glitter delicately highlighting painted finishes of blue, soft greens, creamy yellows and pearl gray. Formal symmetry and balance are important to the style. Benches, daybeds and corner sofas resembling a banquette are often found in the kitchens, offering a comfortable spot to relax. Bulky, overstuffed sofas are out of place in a Swedish Country interior. Wooden ladderback chairs with rush seats, or medallion backed chairs with upholstered seats are also typically Swedish. Chairs could be left natural, painted to resemble more exotic woods, or painted in pale neo-classic tones. Bright peasant reds, blues and greens can also add punch and were popular Arts and Crafts era finishes. Sofas and chairs are generally austere, with minimal upholstery. They often have carved wooden backrests, with padded elbow rests and bolsters added for comfort. White or gray paint with a distressed finish is the most typical look.

Fabrics

Upholstery, window treatments and bedding are usually cotton or linen. Pattern is used sparingly, usually woven checks and stripes, or delicate floral prints. White, blue, pale green, yellow, red and ecru are most typical, with occasional touches of brown or bottle green. One would rarely see a fabric with more than one or two colors against a white or off-white background. Fabrics like toile de jouy, small print calicoes, stripes and checks would look at home in a Swedish Country interior. Scale is not mixed as in a French Country or English Country look, but patterns are of a similar size and scale. Loose calico or linen slipcovers protect fitted upholstery on chairs and settees. Such covers would either be plain or have a simple ruffle around the edges. The simplest muslin swag simply draped above a window instantly creates a classic Swedish Country window treatment. Roller blinds are frequently used in conjunction with muslin swags, fashioned out of plain linen or cotton, or woven stripes or checks on a white or ecru background.

Wallcoverings

Earliest wallcoverings were painted canvas, replacing rich damasks used by the aristocracy. Chinese wall hangings and Chinoiserie wallpapers were highly prized, but most simple Swedish homes relied on painted finishes to decorate and add texture to their walls. Country faux finishes are often wonderfully adventurous. Wild, over-scale marbling was common, as there were few local examples of the real thing to copy. Spattering and stenciling are also typical rustic forms of decorations. Hand painted decorative floral borders and panels with delicate ribbons, swags and wreath motifs are classical Swedish style. Painted lettering, either dates or mottos, were popular Arts and Crafts era adornments.

Accessories

Traditional Swedish style uses few accessories, but their selection and placement is very important. Simplicity, symmetry and usefulness are emphasized. Gleaming silver cutlery and candlesticks, elaborate serving platters and tureens, jugs, bowls and dainty coffee sets, gilded and painted porcelain and traditional blue and white china are all at home in a Swedish Country kitchen. Embroidered linen tablecloths and napkins with clear glassware in simple shapes complete the look. Crystal chandeliers or a ceiling-hung lantern with glass panels would be used for lighting, along with candles placed near mirrors to enhance their effect.

Pale green and yellow beadboard cabinetry, incorporating lots of open shelves, is reminiscent of a Carl Larsson interior. Untreated windows and the use of natural wood tones complete the look in this sunwashed Swedish Country kitchen. ➔

Designed by Kathleen Donohue, CKD, CBD; Photo by Kevin Haislip

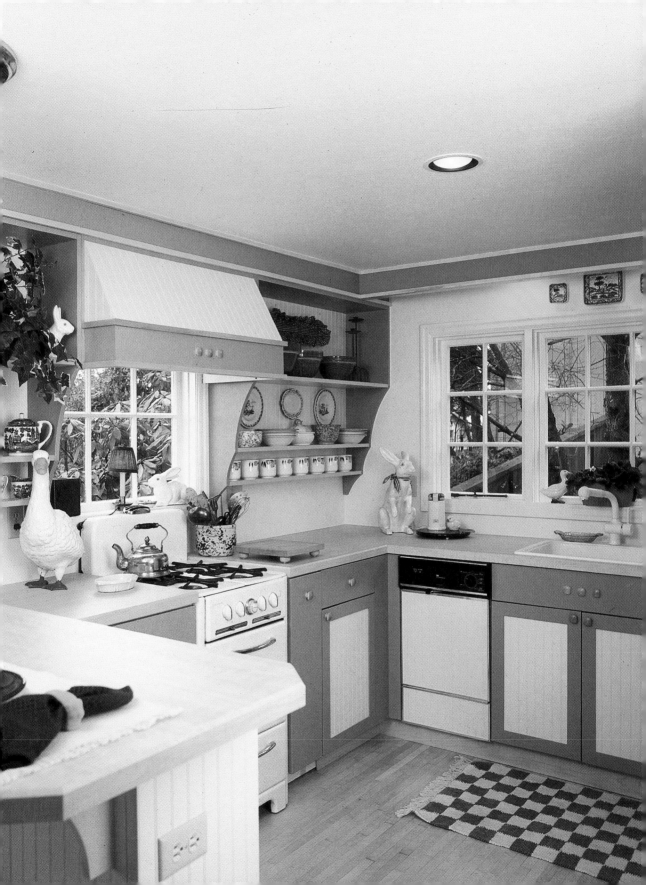

CONCLUSION
MARKETING THEME DESIGN
by Nick Geragi, CKD, CBD, NCIDQ

In today's competitive retail service environment, your ability to understand and implement architectural theme styles can help you to create a niche market. In a time when all in our industry are looking to "*raise the bar on the competition,*" creating theme styles may be a competitive solution. As a tool, making the mental connection between just selling boxes and creating themed kitchens and bathrooms can help us to differentiate ourselves. This becomes a business opportunity for those who can identify the possibilities within the communities they serve. Kitchen and bathroom designers can establish themselves as professionals who can make the connection to the architectural style of the home.

Artfully creating architectural theme styles is not a passive opportunity to be filed away on the bookshelf until you encounter a client who requests a special application of a particular historic style. Rather, it is a diligently crafted specialty that requires self-education and research along with a commitment to investigating all marketing possibilities that exist. Recognize this as a marketing opportunity. A conscious effort must be made to develop the knowledge necessary to create such crafted rooms. If you do not possess an interior design background, get one—teach yourself. Spend time at the library researching theme styles, and architectural and furniture styles. Develop an understanding for the historical timeline of which styles were popular and when. Enroll in a few college courses or local design seminars. Begin a resource library of your own that addresses your market areas, historic roots, or the most popular theme styles of your market segment. Opportunities abound in every region for kitchen and bathroom professionals who deliberately set out to create a name and a niche for themselves.

As you have read in this book, it makes no difference if you are located in the north, south, east or west of North America. In each region, you will find local architectural styles that can be built upon, regardless of the age of the home.

Identifying a Market

But, like many things, creating a niche does not come without some effort. Begin the process by investigating the architectural styles of the homes of your market. Travel through existing neighborhoods, old tract developments and historically zoned districts within your community. Don't forget those condos and townhomes. What do the homes in your market look like, including the new homes being built? Remember, these opportunities are not solely limited to the existence of older neighborhoods. Theme styles are also reflected in new home construction, as was demonstrated in Part I of this book. Throughout, you have even seen how new homes fit established styles, as well as homes that you may have thought had no particular style. Theme styles are not only discovered in the overall architecture of a structure, but also in architectural detailing and furniture styles popular in any given market.

The process for getting involved in this exciting field is simple, but you must be diligent. Visit your local library or historical society and review the local archives of your city, town or province. Research historical events that may have taken place. You may find that historical events often lead to social practices which involve customs and lifestyles that include architectural themes that have developed over a long period of time. Once you have identified the market area that has the potential you are looking for, obtain demographic studies of the potential customer base that lives in that particular area. Find out where they work, average income, the number of family members and other similar facts. The research librarian at your local or county library can help you locate the data. Your local Chamber of Commerce may also be a resource for this type of information.

To further build a reputation as the expert who can create theme styles, attend the local meetings of the historical society or garden club. Participate in their house tours; subscribe to their newsletter and offer to write an article on kitchen and bathroom design. Kitchens and bathrooms are uniquely troublesome rooms to remodel if someone is trying to restore original character in an historic home. The need for modern convenience and updated systems seems to be in contrast, not in harmony, with an historical restoration. The professional kitchen and bathroom designer recognizes this dilemma, and can provide some useful and practical solutions that satisfy both the needs of the modern family for convenience and labor-saving features. Your ability to address these issues is the strength you will want to promote about your services.

Who Can Help

Establish allied partnerships by cultivating business relationships with residential architects, home builders, design/build remodelers, realtors, interior designers, paint stores and antique dealers. Essentially, you want to identify *who* is conducting this type of business, *where* they're doing it, and *how* they're doing it. Offer to collaborate on a kitchen design for an architect's show house or a parade of homes for custom builders, realtors and historical societies. Often, residential developers will have a need for a model home for their newly planned communities. Remember, your customer may not always be the end user, but, may be the allied professional who will require a kitchen or bathroom designer with specialized skills. Create a network among allied professionals where you can refer business to one another, making everyone's role easier by providing allied service and support to each other's clients. Such a network can become a powerful marketing tool.

Taking your niche marketing even further, contact the local design and style editors of your newspapers and magazines. Tell them who you are and what you specialize in. Offer to write an article while providing them with information about projects you have completed and photographed.

Contact your local television or cable station producer. They will often have Sunday special interest and Home and Garden programs for which they are always searching for usable content. These professionals welcome new ideas and slants to a story they can present to their readers and the viewing public.

What Are the Rewards

Besides setting yourself apart from your cabinet competitor, a design focus on theme styles can be financially rewarding. These projects tend to be upper-end jobs sought by more affluent customers, requiring you to employ a consultation fee or a retainer. This customer often recognizes that these projects are complex, so people seeking an integrated statement between the architectural style of their home and its relationship to the home's interior anticipate paying a professional design fee. In most instances, these clients are prequalified and predisposed to completing a project with you, if you can demonstrate your ability to understand the style they desire.

In addition, not only can the specialization of theme styles be financially rewarding to your business, it can give you the opportunity to grow, learn and associate with stimulating and exciting members of the design, building, business, education and media communities. This networking can lead to a recognizable position in your community which, in turn, can earn you more business.

HOW TO RESEARCH AN HISTORIC BUILDING

Who to talk to and how to interview them

Unfortunately, public records fail to cover a great deal of critical information. Much of our heritage is passed on verbally or in family histories or scrapbooks. Frequently, only the most basic information is available from public records or from other documents found at local museums and archives, so it becomes necessary to interview individuals to find out about an historic building. If you run into dead ends, don't despair. As with all detective work, all you need is an inquisitive mind and a bit of determination.

Former occupants and long-time residents can help fill in the gaps left after collecting whatever information can be obtained from public records. But, perhaps more importantly, public records should be used to substantiate and document information garnered from knowledgeable individuals.

Be prepared when you go to interview. If possible, use a tape recorder to ensure accuracy. Prepare a list of questions you would like your interviewee to answer, to prevent allowing either of you to ramble aimlessly; but be flexible, too, as your informant may have valuable information that, at first glance, may not appear to be pertinent. You might want to ask questions first about your interviewee (his/her age, place of origin, occupation, etc.), then proceed on to more general questions about your town or community. Finally, you should ask about the specific house or building you are interested in learning about.

You'll be surprised how often you get your best information where you least expect it. Let your friends and family know about your research. Soon they will be bringing you old photos, newspaper clippings and names of knowledgeable informants.

QUESTIONS TO ASK

About owners, both original and subsequent
- Full name, date of birth, and date of death?
- Place of origin?
- Nationality?
- Occupation?
- Family?
- Civic interests, hobbies, associations, religious affiliations, etc.?

About the building
- Architectural style?
- Date of construction?
- Building technique (balloon framed, post and beam, etc.)?
- Original use and subsequent uses?
- Alterations and additions, including dates of alterations/additions?

Where to go to find answers
- The county clerk's office
- Public library
- Local historical society
- State archive office
- Small, local libraries
- County surveyor's office
- Local or state genealogical associations

Miscellaneous Information

The Sanborn Fire Insurance Company was commissioned to map a number of cities and towns across the U.S., beginning in 1850. The purpose of the maps was to determine potential fire risk. The maps focused on the commercial and industrial sectors. Residences were usually depicted if they surrounded business areas. This was particularly true of earlier maps. Each successive mapping of a town would show more and more land area. Microfilmed black and white copies are often available at Historical Society libraries.

Tips on Putting It All Together

Start with an organized frame of mind and stay organized. Keep all information you collect in one place. Keep notes, photos, clippings and letters in a loose-leaf notebook or scrapbook. This makes it easy to find all your work, and it's a nice way to show family and friends what you've learned about your historic house or building. Remember to thoroughly cite all your sources so that you can retrace your steps if you need more information about something. Write down where you found your information, what page, volume, author, etc. Ask people that you interview about their sources. Good luck!

Terms commonly used in deeds, abstracts and title company records

Consideration - Price paid for the property (In most states, the actual price need not be stated; customary to recite $1 or $10 or "any good and valuable consideration.")

Deed of Bargain and Sale - Conveys the land, not just the grantor's interest. Does not include warranties of title. It is neither a quitclaim or warranty deed.

Grantee - Buyer, second party.

Grantor - Seller, first party (marital status should be clearly stated in deed).

Lien - A hold or claim which one person has on the property of another to secure payment of a debt or other obligation.

Mortgage - A pledge of property to secure the repayment of a debt.

Quitclaim Deed - Purports to convey any interest at the time of sale.

Warranty Deed - Contains covenants of title. Covenants contain certain assurances or guarantees by the grantor that the deed conveys a good and unencumbered title.

Based on a report written by Denyse C. McGriff with the Planning Department, Oregon City, Oregon, 1992.

GLOSSARY

apron. A horizontal board set below the sill of a window or below a horizontal structural member in a piece of furniture.

arch. A curved structural form (usually in segments of a circle) used to span an opening and support a superimposed weight. There are many kinds of arches such as the segmental, elliptical and ogival, which take their names from their geometric forms. Others, such as Tudor, Gothic and Moorish, take their names from the particular time when, or place where, they were used.

architrave. In classic architecture, the lowest section of the entablature. It consisted of a slab or lintel which rested on the column and which supported the frieze, cornice and pediment. In later buildings, a flat molding above any square opening is known as the "architrave."

attic. The portion of an interior wall above the cornice, used in classically inspired architecture.

baluster. A small vertical support for a handrail.

balustrade. Railing for porch, stairway or balcony: includes base, balusters, top railing.

bargeboard. Board, often decorative along roof edge of gable; also called "vergeboard" and "gable trim."

bracket. A flat piece which projects from a wall and forms a support for some weight. Also called a "corbel."

cabriole. S-shaped design of furniture leg, widely used on early 18th century chairs.

capital. The top and most ornamental portion of a column. The capitals of each of the classic orders were stylistically different.

chair rail. The top molding of a dado.

Chinoiserie. A European interpretation of Chinese art, popular from the late 17th to the 19th centuries.

clerestory. Originally the upper story of a Romanesque church which was higher than the surrounding roofs. Now refers to wall space above normal room height; frequently contains window.

coffer. A recessed panel in a ceiling.

column. A vertical, freestanding support for a superstructure. The Greek classic columns were in three styles: the Doric, the Ionic and the Corinthian. The Romans added two more: the Tuscan and the Composite. The proportions and carving on each of these were eventually prescribed. These five have become known as the classic order of architecture.

Corinthian. The latest and most ornate of the classical orders of architecture. The column is slender and usually fluted, the capital elaborately carved with acanthus leaves.

corner post. Vertical boards used to create a finished look at the outside corner of two walls; often designed as a pilaster with ornamental capital and base.

cornice. The moldings which decoratively finish the top of a wall. In classic architecture, the cornice was the top portion of the entablature. It rested on the frieze and supported the pediment.

dado. The woodwork on the lower portion of the walls of a room. It derives from the Italian word for a pedestal and referred to the central portion of the pedestal on which a column rested.

dais. A raised floor in a portion of a room. Originally the word referred to the raised platform at the end of a medieval hall.

Doric. The earliest and plainest of the classical orders. Doric columns usually have no base; the shaft is thick and broadly fluted, the capital spare and unornamented.

damask. Silk or linen fabric, with a lavish textural pattern.

delftware. Tin-glazed earthenware from the Netherlands, traditionally in a blue and white color combination.

dome. A spherical roof.

dormer. A window projecting from a sloping roof.

ebonized. Treated with color to look like real ebony.

entablature. The portion of a classic building which rested on the column and which supported the pediment. It consisted of architrave, frieze and cornice. A complete entablature was used to finish the top portion of a wall, or was used above doors and windows in the most exact, classically inspired periods.

fleur-de-lis. Old French motif that takes the form of a stylized lily or iris.

fretwork. Architectural ornament created with turned members called spindles.

finial. Architectural ornament atop a gable or tower.

frieze. The central portion of an entablature resting on the architrave and supporting the cornice.

gilding. Method of coloring surfaces gold, either by the application of gold leaf or gold paint.

Ionic. One of the classical orders of architecture, characterized by fluted columns and prominent volutes on the capitals.

limewash. Substance composed of slaked lime and water that is used for whitening exterior walls. Also known as whitewash.

linoleum. A floor covering made of compressed cork, ground wood and linseed oil, backed by burlap or strong canvas.

mansard roof. A roof with two slopes, the lower almost vertical to allow extra roof space for the attic rooms.

mantel. The woodwork surrounding a fireplace. The word has now come to refer more especially to the shelf above a fireplace.

marquetry. Decorative veneer composed of inlaid shapes of exotic woods, bone, metal or ivory.

moiré. A fabric or wallpaper, usually silk, that has been treated so that it has a watered or wavelike look.

molding. A narrow-shaped board which is used for a decorative finish to flat boards. In classic architecture, exact names were given to moldings of various sizes and shapes. Some of these were fillet, fascia, ovolo, torus, bead, cavetto, scotia, cyma recta and cyma reversa.

mullion. The slender vertical bar which hold areas of window glass in position. Also known as a "muntin."

newel post. The post into which the handrail of a stairway fits.

panel. The flat board which forms the major portion of interior woodwork. It is held in place by vertical stiles and horizontal rails.

parapet. A low wall surmounting the exterior wall of a building.

parquetry. Intricate patterns, most often geometric, made from small pieces of wood; usually used for flooring.

pediment. The triangular structure in classic architecture which was above the entablature. It is similar to the gable in Nordic architecture. In interior architecture, the pediment was frequently used as a decorative feature. During the 17th century, its pure form was altered to such variations as broken, scroll and segmental pediments.

pilaster. Partial column that projects from a wall.

plinth. The lowest portion of a column, square in shape. In interior architecture, it refers to the rectangular block at the base of a door trim.

portico. Covered entry porch supported by columns or brackets.

quatrefoil. A four-lobed circle or arch formed by cusping.

rail. The horizontal banding which holds a panel in position.

sash. The framing into which the glass of a window is set. The term has come to refer especially to the kind of window frames which slide vertically upon one another.

scroll work. Architectural ornament cut with a scroll or jig saw.

sisal. A natural fiber, used in the manufacture of flooring and rope.

soffit. The underside of a doorway, archway, window, or subordinate architectural member. Used as opposed to "ceiling," which refers to the overhead lining of a room.

stile. The vertical handling which holds a panel board in position.

tracery. An ornamental arrangement of intersecting iron or wood ribwork, usually in the upper part of a Gothic window, forming a pierced pattern. If applied to a solid wall surface, it is known as blind tracery.

transom. The horizontal crossbar of a window or door. The term frequently refers to a small horizontal window above a door.

trefoil. A three-lobed circle or arch formed by cusping.

trim. The wood finish around doors, windows and fireplaces.

trompe l'oeil. A decorative effect, such as a painting of architectural detail or a vista, that gives the illusion of reality.

vault. An arched covering over a corridor.

Vernacular. A term describing humble, often rural architecture, with little or no stylistic pretension, or in a purely regional style, or in a manner based on a naive misunderstanding of high-style architecture.

Vitruvian scroll. A classical frieze ornament, made up of a series of wave-like scrolls, also called a running dog.

wainscot. The name originally referred to wood paneling, held together with tongue-and-groove joints, completely lining a room; now generally refers to paneling which is below the dado.

ziggurat. Architectural pyramidal style with castellated edges, popularly adapted into Art Deco.

RECOMMENDED READING

American Bungalow. 1998. Sierra Madre, CA: John Brinkman Design Offices, Inc.

Cargill, Katrin. 1996. *Swedish style, creating the look.* Pantheon Books.

Cheever, Ellen. 1992. *Beyond the basics...advanced kitchen design.* Hackettstown, NJ: National Kitchen & Bath Association.

Grey, Johnny. 1994. *The art of kitchen design.* Cassell.

Larsson, Carl. 1974. *At home.* G. P. Putnam's & Sons.

MacLachland, Cheryl. 1998. *Bringing France home.* Clarkson Potter, Pub.

Moulin, Pierre, and Pierre LeVec. 1984. *Pierre Deux's French country.* Clarkson N. Potter, Pub.

Old House Interiors. Gloucester, MA: Dovetale Publishers.

Sawyer-Fay, Rebecca. 1995. *Country living; new country kitchens.* Hearst Books.

The Old House Journal Restoration Directory. 1995. Gloucester, MA: Dovetale Publishers.

Turn of the Century Editions. Philmont, NY.

BIBLIOGRAPHY

Baker, John Milnes, AIA. 1994. *American house styles: A concise guide.* New York: W.W. Norton & Co.

Calloway, Stephen, and Elizabeth Cromley, Ed. 1991. *The elements of style; A practical encyclopedia of interior architectural details.* New York: Simon & Schuster.

Calloway, Stephen, and Stephen Jones. 1990. *Style traditions, decorating period interiors.* International Publications Rizzoli.

Del Sordo, Stephen G. 1994. Indoor rain: The shower's short history. *The Old House Journal* (Nov/Dec).

Fisher III, Charles E., Ed. 1989. *The well appointed bath.* Washington, DC: Preservation Press.

Gilliat, Mary. 1990. *Period style.* Little, Brown.

Jackson, Albert, and David Day. 1992. *The complete home restoration manual.* Simon & Schuster.

Jankowski, Wanda. 1993. *Kitchens & baths.* PBC, International, Inc.

Madden, Chris Casson. 1993. *Kitchens.* Clarkson Potter Publishers.

Mayer, Barbara. 1992. *In the arts & crafts style.* Chronical Books.

McAlister, Virginia, and Lee McAlister. 1991. *A field guide to American houses.* Knopf.

McCloud, Kevin. 1990. *Decorative style.* Simon & Schuster.

Miller, Martin, and Judith Miller. 1987. *Period details.* Crown Publishers.

Moss, Roger W. *Lighting for historic buildings.* Washington, DC: Preservation Press.

Nylander, Jane C. 1977. *Fabrics for historic buildings.* Washington, DC: Preservation Press.

Nylander, Richard C. 1983. *Wallpapers for historic buildings.* Washington, DC: Preservation Press.

Plumbing & Mechanical. 1993. The history of plumbing, Parts 1-7, Vol. 10:1. Troy, MI: Business News Publishing Co.

Schwin III, Lawrence. 1994. Decorating old house interiors. Sterling Publishing Company.

Shivers, Natalie. 1990. Walls & molding. Washington, DC: Preservation Press.

Trewby, Mary. 1990. *Classic country and how to achieve it.* Little, Brown & Co.

Von Rosentiel, Helene, and Gail Caskey Winkler. 1988. *Floor coverings for historic buildings.* Washington, DC: The Preservation Press.

Von Zweck, Dina, Ed. 1983. *Woman's Day dictionary of furniture.* Citadel Press.

Index